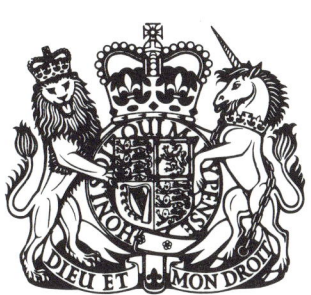

The new NHS
Modern · Dependable

Presented to Parliament by the
Secretary of State for Health
by Command of Her Majesty

December 1997

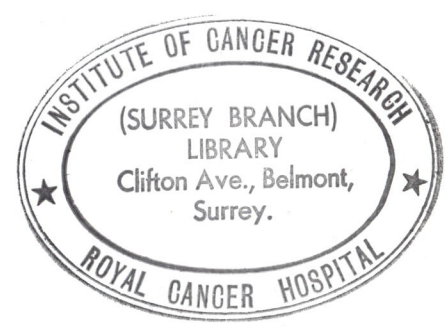

Cm 3807 £12.50

W 225 GRE

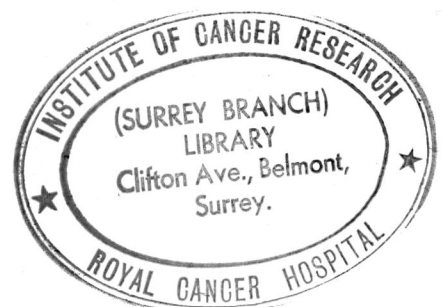

Contents

chapter		page
	Foreword by the Prime Minister	2
1	**A modern and dependable NHS**
there when you need it	4
2	**A new start**
what counts is what works	10
3	**Driving change in the NHS**
quality and efficiency hand in hand	17
4	**Health Authorities**
leading and shaping	24
5	**Primary Care Groups**
going with the grain	32
6	**NHS Trusts**
partnership and performance	44
7	**The national dimension**
a one-nation NHS	55
8	**Measuring progress**
better every year	63
9	**How the money will flow**
from red tape to patient care	68
10	**Making it happen**
rolling out change	76
	Annex
Primary Care Trusts	80
	Glossary	82

Foreword by the Prime Minister

Creating the NHS was the greatest act of modernisation ever achieved by a Labour Government. It banished the fear of becoming ill that had for years blighted the lives of millions of people. But I know that one of the main reasons people elected a new Government on May 1st was their concern that the NHS was failing them and their families. In my contract with the people of Britain I promised that we would rebuild the NHS. We have already made a start. The Government is putting an extra £1.5 billion into the health service during the course of this year and next. More money is going into improving breast cancer and children's services. And new hospitals are being built. The NHS will get better every year so that it once again delivers dependable, high quality care - based on need, not ability to pay.

This White Paper marks a turning point for the NHS. It replaces the internal market with integrated care. We are saving £1 billion of red tape and putting that money into frontline patient care. For the first time the need to ensure that high quality care is spread throughout the service will be taken seriously. National standards of care will be guaranteed. There will be easier and swifter access to the NHS when you need it. Our approach combines efficiency and quality with a belief in fairness and partnership.

1948 public information leaflet

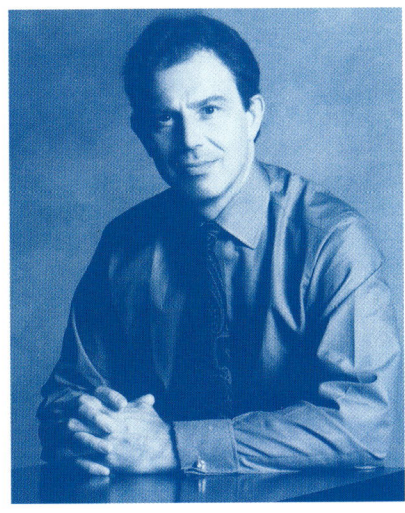

As we approach the fiftieth anniversary of the NHS, it is time to reflect on the huge achievements of the NHS. But in a changing world no organisation, however great, can stand still. The NHS needs to modernise in order to meet the demands of today's public. This White Paper begins a process of modernisation. The NHS will start to provide new and better services to the public. For example, a nurse-led helpline to provide advice round the clock. And new technology that links GP surgeries to any specialist centre in the country.

In short, I want the NHS to take a big step forward and become a modern and dependable service that is once more the envy of the world.

Of course we must get the funding right. The Government has already put large extra sums into the NHS, and will raise spending in real terms every year. With that money comes a responsibility within the service to change. To produce better care. Care when you need it. Care of uniformly high standards.

It is a big challenge but I am confident that with the support of the public, the dedication of NHS staff and the backing of the Government we can again create an NHS that is truly a beacon to the world.

Tony Blair

Tony Blair

1 Key themes

- *£1 billion from red tape into patient care*
- *NHS Direct – 24-hour nurse helpline*
- *NHS information superhighway*
- *guaranteed fast-track cancer services*

A modern and dependable NHS
there when you need it

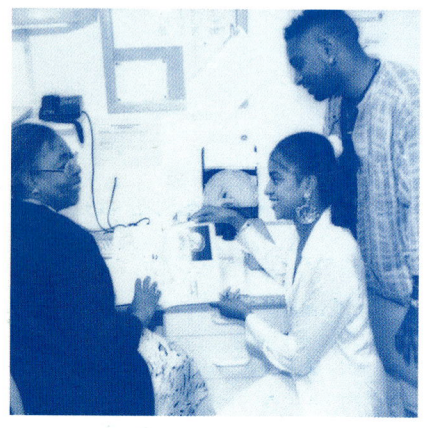

The new NHS

1.1 The Government is committed to giving the people of this country the best system of health care in the world. At its best the National Health Service is the envy of the world. But often it takes too long for patients to get treated. Quality is variable. And NHS staff feel too much of their time and effort is diverted from treating patients into pushing paper. This White Paper explains how the Government, working with those one million staff, will build a modern and dependable health service fit for the twenty first century. A **national** health service which offers people prompt high quality treatment and care when and where they need it. An NHS that does not just treat people when they are ill but works with others to improve health and reduce health inequalities.

'prompt high quality treatment and care'

1.2 Achieving this vision means we have to change our approach to tackling ill-health and inequality. The Government will ensure the NHS works locally with those who provide social care, housing, education and employment, just as the Government itself will work nationally across Whitehall to bring about lasting improvements in the public's health. The forthcoming Green Paper *Our Healthier Nation* will outline this strategy in more detail.

1.3 But we also have to change the way that the NHS itself is run. The introduction of the internal market by the previous Government prevented the health service from properly focusing on the needs of patients. It wasted resources administering competition between hospitals. This White Paper sets out how the internal market will be replaced by a system we have called 'integrated care', based on partnership and driven by performance. It forms the basis for a ten year programme to renew and improve the NHS through evolutionary change rather than organisational upheaval. These changes will build on what has worked, but discard what has failed.

> *'integrated care based on partnership and driven by performance'*

1.4 The needs of patients will be central to the new system. Abolishing the internal market will enable health professionals to focus on patients, making the NHS better every year. Individual patients, who too often have been passed from pillar to post between competing agencies, will get access to an integrated system of care that is quick and reliable. Local doctors and nurses, who best understand patients' needs, will shape local services. Patients will be guaranteed national standards of excellence so that they can have confidence in the quality of the services they receive. There will be new incentives and new sanctions to improve quality and efficiency. Frontline patient services will be backed by more investment and better technology. These changes will bring a more responsive and dependable service to every community in England.

> *'more investment and better technology'*

1.5 The Government has committed itself anew to the historic principle of the NHS: that if you are ill or injured there will be a national health service there to help; and access to it will be based on need and need alone - not on your ability to pay, or on who your GP happens to be or on where you live. The NHS has stood the test of time for fifty years. But the Government was elected with a mandate to change the NHS for the better. This White Paper will modernise the NHS so that it is prepared for the next fifty years.

> **The Government's Commitment**
>
> If you are ill or injured there will be a national health service there to help: and access to it will be based on need and need alone - not on your ability to pay, or on who your GP happens to be or on where you live.

1.6 The speed of change in science and medicine and the potential of modern information and communication systems require the NHS to embrace change. A modern and dependable national health service will capture developments in modern medicine and information technology. It will be built around the needs of people, not of institutions and it will provide prompt reliable care. It will learn from those at the leading edge of good practice and will make the best available to all.

1.7 Realising this vision of a modern and dependable NHS means providing:

- **at home:** easier and faster **advice and information** for people about health, illness and the NHS so that they are better able to care for themselves and their families

- **in the community: swift advice and treatment in local surgeries and health centres** with family doctors and community nurses working alongside other health and social care staff to provide a wide range of services on the spot

- **in hospital: prompt access to specialist services** linked to local surgeries and health centres so that entry, treatment and care are seamless and quick.

1.8 Some of these developments are already available to some patients, but not everywhere. The Government wants to see them available to all as part and parcel of the new NHS.

'NHS Direct, a new 24 hour telephone advice line staffed by nurses'

1.9 This is an ambitious programme which cannot happen overnight. It will be achieved over ten years with demonstrable improvements each year. We have already made a start. The process of modernisation began on May 2nd, the day after the election. Since then the worst excesses of the internal market have been tackled and extra resources devoted to patient care.

1.10 The changes in this White Paper will take forward the modernisation of the NHS. The Government has pledged to cut waiting lists for hospital treatment. By the end of this Parliament we will have done so. But more needs to be done at all levels if the vision is to be made real. Three developments will symbolise our new approach.

1.11 **At home:** we will provide easier and faster advice and information through NHS Direct, a new **24 hour telephone advice line** staffed by nurses. We will pilot this through three care and advice helplines to begin in March 1998. The whole country will be covered by 2000.

'connecting every GP surgery and hospital to the NHS's own information superhighway'

1.12 **In the community:** patients will benefit from quicker test results, up-to-date specialist advice in the doctor's surgery and on-line booking of out-patient appointments, when we **connect every GP surgery and hospital to NHSnet**, the NHS's own information superhighway. It could also mean less waiting for prescriptions in the pharmacy because of electronic links between GPs and pharmacists. As a first step, by the end of 1998 demonstration sites will be established in every Region to pilot how the NHSnet can be used to bring direct benefits to patients. As a second step, by the end of 1999 all computerised GP surgeries will be able to receive some hospital test results over NHSnet. By 2002, these services will be available across the country.

1.13 **In hospital:** we will improve prompt **access to specialist services** so that everyone with suspected cancer will be able to see a specialist within two weeks of their GP deciding they need to be seen urgently and requesting an appointment. We will guarantee these arrangements for everyone with suspected breast cancer by April 1999 and for all other cases of suspected cancer by 2000.

1.14 These developments, along with the pledge to cut waiting lists, will chart progress to a quicker and more responsive NHS. They will demonstrate that services to patients are getting better every year.

'everyone with suspected cancer will be able to see a specialist within two weeks'

The Challenge

1.15 Some say that this vision is not just ambitious, but unachievable; that tailoring the NHS to meet the needs of individual patients is simply beyond its capacity. They believe that the NHS is being overwhelmed by three big pressures: growing public expectations, medical advances and demographic changes.

1.16 It is certainly true that people do expect more, especially in speed of service and range of treatment. The pace of medical advance does create demands for new techniques to be assimilated and spread. And rising numbers of elderly people are looking to the NHS for a level of active treatment which would have been unimaginable in the past.

1.17 Those who argue that the NHS cannot accommodate these pressures say that it will need huge increases in taxation, a move to a charge-based service, or radical restrictions in patient care.

1.18 The Government rejects this analysis. So do the public. The recent British Social Attitudes Survey showed that three-quarters of people want the NHS to remain a universal health service. Two-thirds believe that health care should be available to all on the basis of need, not ability to pay. Nor are the arguments in favour of rationing or charging convincing.

1.19 First, the pressures on the NHS are exaggerated. Indeed they have always been exaggerated. It was Nye Bevan who noted some 50 years ago that "expectations will always exceed capacity". Rising public expectations should be channelled into shaping services to make them more responsive to the needs and preferences of the

'tailoring the NHS to meet the needs of individual patients'

A modern and dependable NHS

> *'the health service is a strong and resilient organisation'*

people who use them. Many women, for example, have welcomed the opportunity to plan the arrangements for the birth of their child with midwives as well as doctors. Our new NHS Charter will balance the patient's rights of access to NHS services with their responsibility to use services wisely.

1.20 The health service is a strong and resilient organisation. It has risen to daunting challenges over the past ten years, such as AIDS, more operations for coronary artery bypass grafts, and new drugs for stomach ulcers. Of course many new problems lie ahead but not all will increase the health care bill. As technology advances, allowing less invasive and hence cheaper treatments, costs in certain areas will be reduced. Heart catheters, in some cases, could increasingly replace bypass grafts, for example, or more day surgery could reduce expensive inpatient care. Taking a longer term view, the Government's new emphasis on improving public health and tackling inequalities will also help.

Demographic pressures

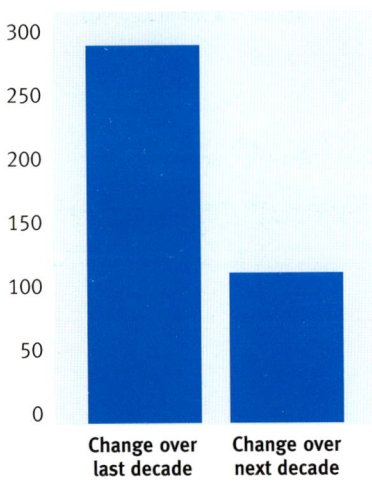

Age 85 & over
thousands

1.21 Likewise demographic pressures can be overstated. Over the next decade the NHS expects to provide services for an extra 100,000 people aged 85 and over; but that is just one-third of the increase that it has coped with over the last decade.

1.22 Second, the choice posed between unaffordable levels of funding or charges and rationing is a false dilemma. No-one denies that the NHS needs more money every year. With this Government the health service will get it. We are committed to increasing spending on the NHS in real terms every year. But there are three other changes that will ensure better value for money in the NHS:

- the NHS needs to make **better use of its resources.** The internal market has driven up administrative costs. The Government's changes will reduce costs by £1 billion over the lifetime of the current Parliament. Fragmentation in decision-making has lost the NHS the cost advantages that collaboration can bring. Cooperation and efficiency go hand in glove. The proposals in this White Paper will produce a new drive on efficiency, quality and performance in the NHS

> *'we are committed to increasing spending on the NHS in real terms every year'*

- the NHS should **harness new developments** rather than be driven by them. There are already mechanisms in place to evaluate new technologies, and to measure the clinical and cost-effectiveness of treatments. NHS funded research has, for example, already shown that universal screening for prostate cancer would not be worthwhile and new approaches to prescribing in primary care are helping to deliver better care at lower cost. But the take-up of research findings on clinical and cost-effectiveness is uneven and unsystematic. For example there are big variations in day case rates. In order to sustain the NHS, while making it both modern and dependable, this White Paper proposes a new drive for quality. Two new national bodies will lead rigorous assessment of clinical and cost-effective treatments and will ensure good practice is adopted locally

- decisions about how best to use resources for patient care are best made by those who treat patients - and this principle is at the heart of the proposals in this White Paper. For the first time in the history of the NHS the Government will align clinical and financial responsibility to give all the professionals who make prescribing and referring decisions the opportunity to make financial decisions in the best interests of their patients. That will better attune local services to meet local needs. But the Government will set a framework of national standards and will monitor performance to ensure consistency and fairness.

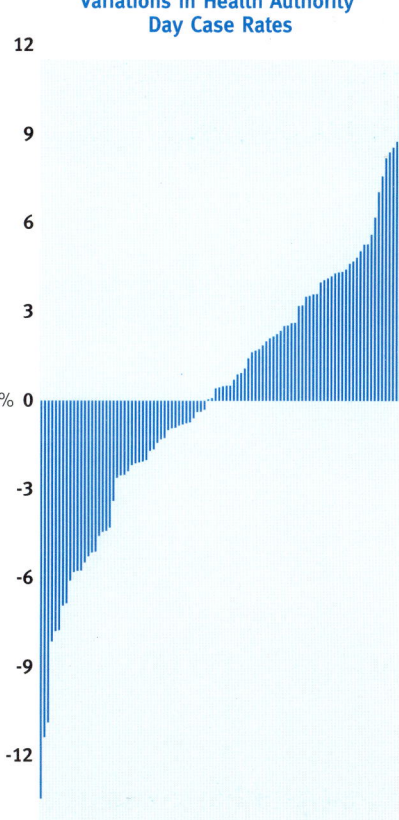

Variations in Health Authority Day Case Rates

On average 60% of patients from waiting lists were treated as day cases in 1996/97

'the health of the economy depends on the health of the NHS'

1.23 There is another reason why it makes sense to sustain the NHS as a universal service. The health of the economy depends on the health of the NHS. It helps ensure a healthy workforce. But it does much more besides. The NHS funded through general taxation is the fairest and most efficient way of providing health care for the population at large. Systems in other countries cost more, are less fair, and deliver little overall extra benefit. The cost-effectiveness of the NHS helps to reduce the tax burden to well below the European Union average, encouraging investment and strengthening incentives to work and save. The alternatives - rationing or a 'charge-based' system - would dissipate these advantages.

1.24 But it is clear there are tough choices facing the NHS. It has to improve its performance if it is to deliver the sort of services patients need. There will have to be big gains in quality and big gains in efficiency across the whole NHS. The two go together. They will bring about marked improvements in services to patients over the next ten years. This White Paper spells out how the NHS will meet that challenge. There can be no standing still. The next two chapters outline the Government's approach. The subsequent chapters set out the arrangements in detail, showing how they will work in practice. They are the means to deliver a modern and dependable health care system that will once again lead the world. A new NHS for a new century.

2 Key themes

- *the third way*
- *keeping what works*
- *discarding what has failed*

A new start
what counts is what works

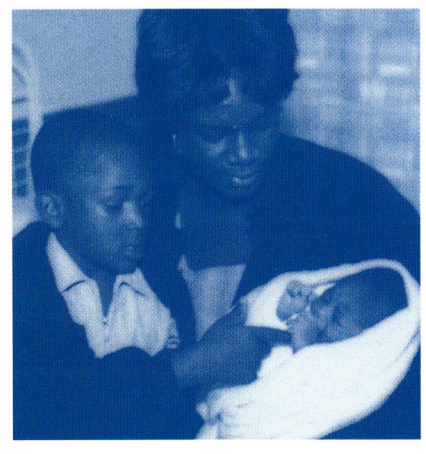

The third way

2.1 In paving the way for the new NHS the Government is committed to building on what has worked, but discarding what has failed. There will be no return to the old centralised command and control systems of the 1970s. That approach stifled innovation and put the needs of institutions ahead of the needs of patients. But nor will there be a continuation of the divisive internal market system of the 1990s. That approach which was intended to make the NHS more efficient ended up fragmenting decision-making and distorting incentives to such an extent that unfairness and bureaucracy became its defining features.

2.2 Instead there will be a 'third way' of running the NHS - a system based on partnership and driven by performance. It will go with the grain of recent efforts by NHS staff to overcome the obstacles of the internal market. Increasingly those working in primary care, NHS Trusts and Health Authorities have tried to move away from outright competition towards a more collaborative approach. Inevitably, however, these efforts have been only partially successful and their benefits have not as yet been extended to patients in all parts of the country.

2.3 This White Paper will put that right. It builds on the extensive discussions we have held with a wide range of NHS staff and organisations. It will develop this more collaborative approach into a new system for the whole NHS. It will neither be the model from the late 1970s nor the model from the early 1990s. It will be a new model for a new century.

'a new model for a new century'

Six key principles

2.4 Six important principles underlie the changes we are now proposing:

- first, to renew the NHS as a genuinely **national** service. Patients will get fair access to consistently high quality, prompt and accessible services right across the country

- but second, to make the delivery of healthcare against these new national standards a matter of **local** responsibility. Local doctors and nurses who are in the best position to know what patients need will be in the driving seat in shaping services

- third, to get the NHS to work in **partnership**. By breaking down organisational barriers and forging stronger links with Local Authorities, the needs of the patient will be put at the centre of the care process

- but fourth, to drive **efficiency** through a more rigorous approach to performance and by cutting bureaucracy, so that every pound in the NHS is spent to maximise the care for patients

- fifth, to shift the focus onto quality of care so that **excellence** is guaranteed to all patients, and quality becomes the driving force for decision-making at every level of the service

- and sixth, to rebuild **public confidence** in the NHS as a public service, accountable to patients, open to the public and shaped by their views.

'local doctors and nurses in the driving seat'

'excellence guaranteed to all patients'

Keeping what works

2.5 There are some sound foundations on which the new NHS can be built. Not everything about the old system was bad. This Government believes that what counts is what works. If something is working effectively then it should not be discarded purely for the sake of it. The new system will go with the grain of the best of these developments.

A new start

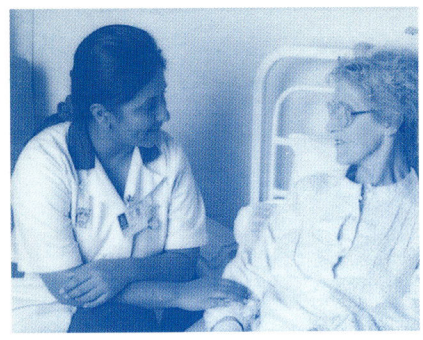

'the needs of patients not the needs of institutions will be at the heart of the new NHS'

Primary and Community Services

Most people look first to their family doctor or local pharmacist for advice on health matters. Dentists, optometrists and ophthalmic medical practitioners also provide essential care to meet everyday needs.
Community health service staff offer a range of services for people wherever they are, in their homes, schools, clinics and even in the streets. These services include health visiting, school nursing, chiropody, occupational, speech and language therapy. Services such as district nursing, community psychiatric nursing and physiotherapy can enable people with short or long term disability to be cared for in their own homes. Other specialist staff such as midwives provide care across hospital and community settings.

2.6 The Government will retain the **separation between the planning of hospital care and its provision.** This is the best way to put into practice the new emphasis on improving health and on meeting the healthcare needs of the whole community. By empowering local doctors, nurses and Health Authorities to plan services we will ensure that the local NHS is built around the needs of patients. Hospitals and other agencies providing services will have a hand in shaping those plans but their primary duty will be to meet patients' requirements for high quality and easily accessible services. The needs of patients not the needs of institutions will be at the heart of the new NHS.

2.7 The Government will also build on the increasingly **important role of primary care** in the NHS. Most of the contact that patients have with the NHS is through a primary care professional such as a community nurse or a family doctor. They are best placed to understand their patients' needs as a whole and to identify ways of making local services more responsive. Family doctors who have been involved in commissioning services (either as fundholders, or through multifunds, locality commissioning or the total purchasing model) have welcomed the chance to influence the use of resources to improve patient care. The Government wishes to build on these approaches, ensuring that all patients, rather than just some, are able to benefit.

2.8 Finally, the Government recognises the intrinsic strength of **decentralising responsibility for operational management.** By giving NHS Trusts control over key decisions they can improve local services for patients. The Government will build on this principle and let NHS Trusts help shape the locally agreed framework which will determine how NHS services develop. In the future the approach will be interdependence rather than independence.

Discarding what has failed

2.9 The internal market was a misconceived attempt to tackle the pressures facing the NHS. It has been an obstacle to the necessary modernisation of the health service. It created more problems than it solved. That is why the Government is abolishing it.

Ending fragmentation

2.10 The internal market split responsibility for planning, funding and delivering healthcare between 100 Health Authorities, around 3,500 GP fundholders (representing half of GP practices) and over 400 NHS Trusts. There was little strategic coordination. A fragmented NHS has been poorly placed to tackle the crucial issue of better integration across health and social care. People with multiple needs have found themselves passed from pillar to post inside a system in which individual organisations were forced to work to their own agendas rather than the needs of individual patients.

2.11 To overcome this fragmentation, in the new NHS all those charged with planning and providing health and social care services for patients will work to a jointly agreed local Health Improvement Programme. This will govern the actions of all the parts of the local NHS to ensure consistency and coordination. It will also make clear the responsibilities of the NHS and local authorities for working together to improve health.

> **Health Improvement Programme**
>
> An action programme led by the Health Authority to improve health and healthcare locally will involve NHS Trusts, Primary Care Groups and other primary care professionals, working in partnership with the local authority and other local interests. See chapter 4.

Ending unfairness

2.12 The internal market created competition for patients. In the process it created unfairness for patients. Some family doctors were able to get a better deal for their patients, for financial rather than clinical reasons. Staff morale has been eroded by an emphasis on competitive values, at odds with the ethos of fairness that is intrinsic to the NHS and its professions. Hospital clinicians have felt disempowered as they have been deliberately pitted against each other and against primary care. The family doctor community has been divided in two, almost equally split between GP fundholders and non-fundholders.

'cooperation will replace competition'

2.13 In the new NHS patients will be treated according to need and need alone. Cooperation will replace competition. GPs and community nurses will work together in Primary Care Groups. Hospital clinicians will have a say in developing local Health Improvement Programmes.

Ending distortion

2.14 The market forced NHS organisations to compete against each other even when it would have made better sense to cooperate. Some were

A new start

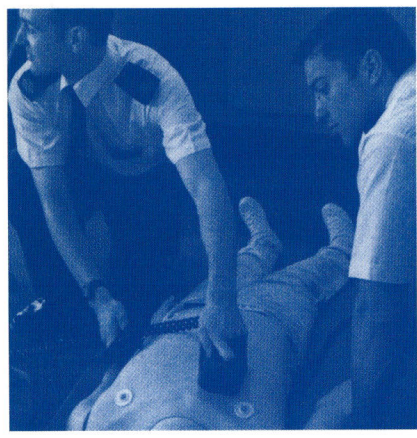

'best practice available to patients wherever they live'

unwilling to share best practice that might benefit a wider range of patients in case they forfeited competitive advantage. Quality has been at best variable.

2.15 In the new NHS, there will be new mechanisms to share best practice so that it becomes available to patients wherever they live. A new national performance framework for ensuring high performance and quality will, over time, tackle variable standards of service.

Ending inefficiency

2.16 Under the internal market, the Purchaser Efficiency Index was the only real measure of performance. But it distorted priorities and - to the universal frustration of NHS staff - institutionalised perverse incentives which got in the way of providing efficient, effective, high quality services. In addition, budgets for emergency care, waiting list surgery and drug treatments were artificially divided, reducing flexibility.

2.17 In the new NHS, the Purchaser Efficiency Index will be replaced by better measures of real efficiency as part of a broader set of performance measures. They will assess the NHS against the things which count most for patients, including the costs and results of treatment and care. National reference costs will allow NHS Trusts to benchmark their performance. And partitioned budgets will be unified so that total resources can be matched locally against the needs of patients, ensuring more efficient and appropriate care.

Ending bureaucracy

2.18 The internal market sent administrative costs soaring to unsustainable levels. In recent years effort and resources have been diverted from improving patient services. With so many players on the field, transaction costs in the NHS inevitably spiralled.

2.19 This White Paper will cap management costs and cut the number of commissioning bodies from around 3,600 to as few as 500. The Government has already taken steps to reduce transaction costs and along with the changes in this White Paper £1 billion in administration will be saved over the lifetime of this Parliament for investment in patient services.

Internal market bureaucracy

Evidence shows that:

- one fundholder with a contract worth £150,000 received 1,000 pieces of paper per year

- a Health Authority in the south processed 60,000 invoices per year representing 8% of its healthcare budget

- an inner city Trust contracted with over 900 funds and sent out 40,000 invoices per year

Ending instability

2.20 The internal market forced NHS Trusts to compete for contracts that at best lasted a year and at worst were agreed on a day-to-day basis. Such short-term instability placed a constant focus on shoring up the status quo rather than creating the space to plan and implement major improvement.

2.21 This White Paper will scrap annual contracts. Instead, the new NHS will work on the basis of longer-term three and in some cases five year funding agreements that will allow clinicians and managers to focus on ways of improving care.

Ending secrecy

2.22 Under the internal market hospitals became 'self-governing trusts' run as businesses, focused on finance, and required to compete with each other for short-term contracts. Increasingly NHS Trust Boards meeting in secret made it hard for local people to find out what their local hospital was planning and how it was performing. GP fundholders could make significant purchasing decisions without reference to the local community.

2.23 In the new NHS, all NHS Trusts will be required to open up their board meetings to the public. They will have new statutory duties on quality and on working in partnership with others. Comparative information on NHS Trust performance will be published. Openness and public involvement will be key features of all parts of the new NHS.

2.24 These developments will place the traditional values of the NHS into a modern setting. They will be backed by the Government's commitment to extra investment in the NHS, year on year. But that extra money has to produce major gains in quality and efficiency. Otherwise the health service will simply not keep pace with the needs of the public it is there to serve. The NHS has to make better use of its resources to ensure that it delivers better, more responsive services for patients everywhere. It has to share best practice and eliminate poor performance so that patients have a guarantee of excellence. The next chapter describes how quality and efficiency will be instilled in all parts of the NHS.

Unacceptable variations

At its best, the NHS leads the world. But the degree of local variation means that individual patients cannot be sure of receiving that best:

- the death rate from coronary heart disease in people younger than 65 is almost three times higher in Manchester than in West Surrey

- emergency readmissions to hospital are 70% higher in one area than in another

- the proportion of women aged 25-64 screened for cervical cancer varies from 67% to 93% in different areas

- the number of hip replacements in over 65s varies from 10 to 51 per 10,000 of the population

- the number of outpatients seen within 13 weeks of written GP referral varies from 71% to 98%

- the number of outpatients admitted for elective treatment who have waited less than 3 months since a decision to admit varies from 56% to 82%

- the percentage of drugs prescribed generically varies from below 50% to almost 70%

- the percentage of consultant episodes carried out as day cases varies from below 50% to almost 70%.

How we are replacing the Internal Market with Integrated Care

Internal Market	Integrated Care
Fragmented responsibility between 4,000 NHS bodies. Little strategic planning. Patients passed from pillar to post	Health Improvement Programmes jointly agreed by all who are charged with planning or providing health and social care
Competition between hospitals. Some GPs get better service for their patients at the expense of others. Hospital clinicians disempowered	Patients treated according to need, not who their GP is, or where they live. Co-operation will replace competition. Hospital clinicians involved
Competition prevented sharing of best practice, to protect 'competitive advantage'. Variable quality	New mechanisms to share best practice. New performance framework to tackle variable standards of quality
Perverse incentives of Efficiency Index, distorting priorities, and getting in the way of real efficiency, effectiveness and quality. Artificially partitioned budgets	Efficiency Index replaced by new reference costs. Broader set of performance measures. Budgets unified for maximum flexibility and efficiency
Soaring administrative costs, diverting effort from improving patient services. High numbers of invoices and high transaction costs	Management costs capped. Number of commissioning bodies cut from 3,600 to 500. Transaction costs cut
Short term contracts, focusing on cost and volume. Incentive on each NHS Trust to lever up volume to meet financial targets rather than work across organisational boundaries	Longer term service agreements linked to quality improvements. NHS Trusts share responsibility for appropriate service usage
NHS Trusts run as secretive commercial businesses. Unrepresentative boards. Principal legal duty on finance	NHS Trusts with representative boards and end to secrecy. New legal duties on quality and partnership

Key themes

- *raising quality standards*
- *increasing efficiency*
- *driving performance*
- *new roles and responsibilities*

3

Driving change in the NHS
quality and efficiency hand in hand

3.1 The new NHS will work as one. There will be clear roles and responsibilities for each part of the health service. It will work to new standards of quality and efficiency that will guarantee better services for patients. The new NHS will be performance driven. This chapter summarises the main features of the new system and describes the key role each part of the NHS will play. Later chapters give greater detail.

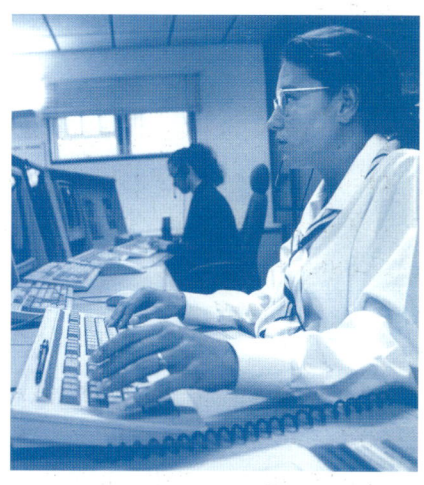

Driving quality

3.2 The new NHS will have quality at its heart. Without it there is unfairness. Every patient who is treated in the NHS wants to know that they can rely on receiving high quality care when they need it. Every part of the NHS, and everyone who works in it, should take responsibility for working to improve quality. This must be quality in its broadest sense: doing the right things, at the right time, for the right people, and doing them right - first time. And it must be the quality of the patient's experience as well as the clinical result - quality measured in terms of prompt access, good relationships and efficient administration.

'raising standards and ensuring consistency'

3.3 There is much to build on. Clearing away the distraction of the market will help staff get attention back where it counts. But new and systematic action is needed, to raise standards and ensure consistency. There have been some serious lapses in quality. When they have occurred they have harmed individual patients and dented public confidence.

3.4 This White Paper sets out three areas for action to drive quality into all parts of the NHS: **national standards and guidelines** for services and treatments; **local measures** to enable NHS staff to take responsibility for improving quality; and a new **organisation to address shortcomings**.

3.5 Nationally there will be:

- new evidence-based **National Service Frameworks** to help ensure consistent access to services and quality of care right across the country

- a new **National Institute for Clinical Excellence** to give a strong lead on clinical and cost-effectiveness, drawing up new guidelines and ensuring they reach all parts of the health service.

> **National Service Frameworks**
>
> National Service Frameworks will bring together the best evidence of clinical and cost-effectiveness, with the views of service users, to determine the best ways of providing particular services. See also chapter 7.

3.6 Locally there will be:

- teams of **local GPs and community nurses** working together in new Primary Care Groups to shape services for patients, concentrating on the things which really count - prompt, accessible, seamless care delivered to a high standard

- explicit quality standards in local **service agreements** between Health Authorities, Primary Care Groups and NHS Trusts, reflecting national standards and targets

- a new system of **clinical governance** in NHS Trusts and primary care to ensure that clinical standards are met, and that processes are in place to ensure continuous improvement, backed by a new **statutory duty** for quality in NHS Trusts.

'a new statutory duty for quality'

3.7 A new **Commission for Health Improvement** will be established to support and oversee the quality of clinical services at local level, and to tackle shortcomings. It will be able to intervene where necessary. The Secretary of State will also have reserve powers to intervene directly when a problem has not been gripped.

Driving efficiency

3.8 Efficiency and quality should go hand in hand. Both are essential in a modern and dependable NHS. Both are essential to fairness. Patients suffer if resources are not used efficiently or to best effect, just as they suffer if quality standards vary. This White Paper outlines five ways to ensure the NHS delivers universally high standards in the efficient and effective use of resources and in financial discipline.

3.9 First, **clinical and financial responsibility will be aligned**. Primary Care Groups will be able to take devolved responsibility for a **single unified budget** covering most aspects of care so that they can get the best fit between resources and need. It will provide local family doctors and community nurses with maximum freedom to use the resources available to the benefit of patients, with efficiency incentives at both Group and practice level.

3.10 Second, **management costs will be capped** in Health Authorities and Primary Care Groups. The Government will also continue to bear down on NHS Trust management costs, benchmarking performance. This approach will get the maximum NHS resources into frontline patient services.

3.11 Third, the Government will develop a national schedule of **'reference costs'** which will itemise what individual treatments across the NHS cost. By requiring NHS Trusts to publish and benchmark their own costs on the same basis, the new arrangements will give Health Authorities, Primary Care Groups and the NHS Executive a strong lever with which to tackle inefficiency.

3.12 Fourth, there will be **clear incentives** to improve performance and efficiency. Health Authorities which perform well will be eligible for extra cash. NHS Trusts and Primary Care Groups will be able to use savings from longer term agreements to improve services for patients.

3.13 Fifth, there will be **clear sanctions** when performance and efficiency are not up to standard. Health Authorities will be able to withdraw freedoms from Primary Care Groups. They, in turn, will have a range of new powers to lever up standards and efficiency at local NHS Trusts and as a last resort will be able to change provider if, over time, performance does not meet the required standard. And the NHS Executive will be able directly to intervene to rectify poor performance in any part of the NHS.

> **Single unified budget**
>
> For the first time funding for all hospital and community services, prescribing and general practice infrastructure will be brought together into a single stream at Health Authority and Primary Care Group level.

'management costs will be capped'

Bringing quality and efficiency together

3.14 The Government will bring these developments together in a new *'the pursuit of quality and efficiency must go together if the NHS is to deliver the best for patients'*

approach to measuring the performance of the NHS and holding it to account. Experience shows that the way in which performance is measured directly affects how the NHS acts; the wrong measures produce the wrong results. New arrangements will concentrate on measuring what really counts for patients through a new Performance Framework. It will focus on more rounded measures - health improvement, fairer access to services, better quality and outcomes of care and the views of patients - as well as real efficiency gains.

3.15 This new approach will demonstrate how the pursuit of quality and efficiency must go together if the NHS is to deliver the best for patients. The new Performance Framework will be used to get all parts of the NHS working together to ensure that both the local health service and the health of local people are getting demonstrably better every year.

New information technology - supporting quality and efficiency

A modern and dependable NHS needs to be supported by accurate and up-to-date information and information technology. In recent years, information technology in the NHS has been focused on supporting the transaction processes of the internal market. This has been at the expense of realising the potential of IT to support frontline staff in delivering benefits for patients. In 1998, the Government will publish a new Information Management and Technology Strategy for the NHS which will harness the enormous potential benefits of IT to support the drive for quality and efficiency in the NHS by:

- making patient records electronically available when they're needed
- using the NHSnet and the Internet to bring patients quicker test results, on-line booking of appointments and up-to-date specialist advice
- enabling accurate information about finance and performance to be available promptly
- providing knowledge about health, illness and best treatment practice to the public through the Internet and emerging public access media (e.g. digital TV)
- developing telemedicine to ensure specialist skills are available to all parts of the country

There will be robust safeguards to protect patients' confidentiality and privacy. The aim will be to create a powerful alliance between knowledgeable patients advised by knowledgeable professionals as a means of improving health and healthcare.

Figure 1: **Financing and accountability arrangements in the new NHS compared with the old**

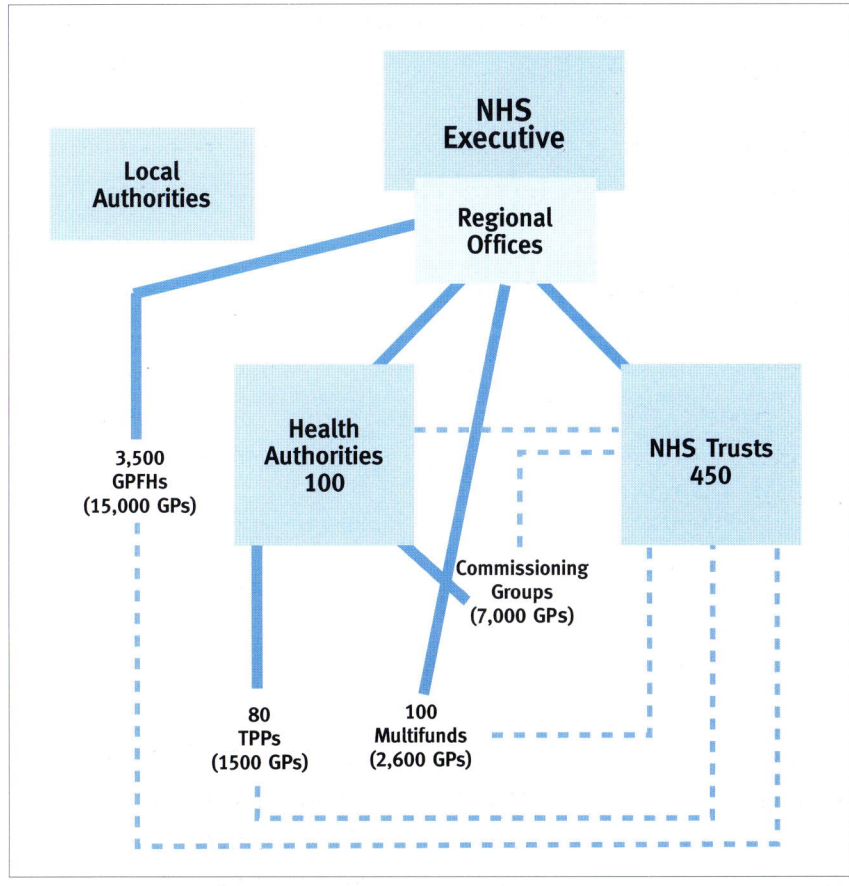

The old NHS

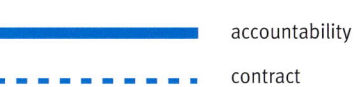

——————— accountability
- - - - - - - - contract

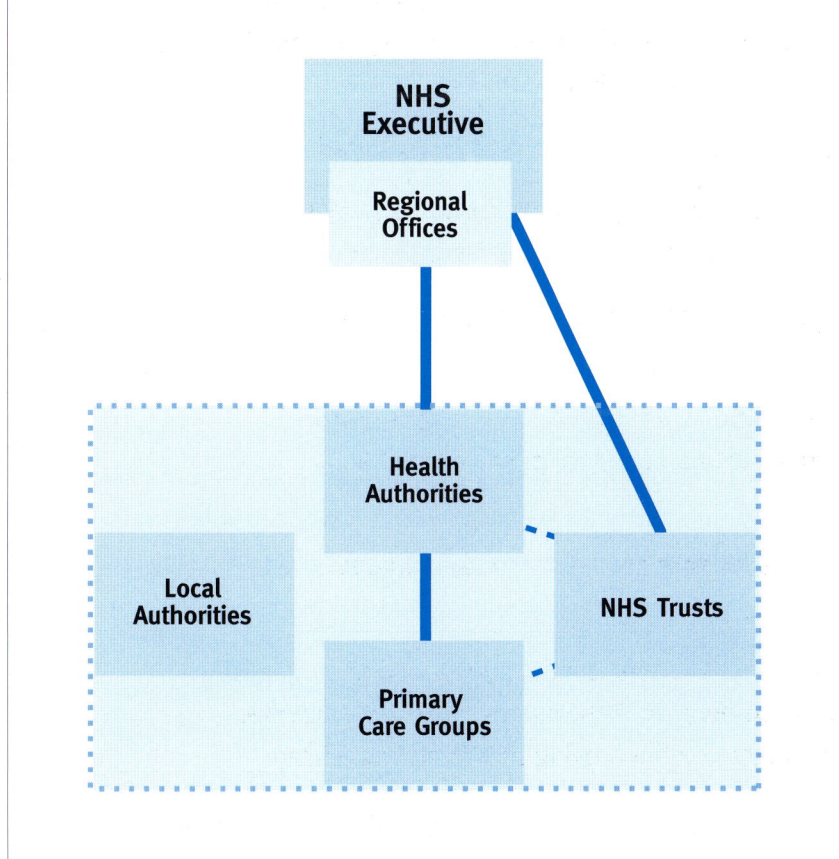

The new NHS

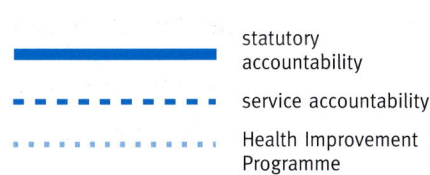

——————— statutory accountability
- - - - - - - - service accountability
············· Health Improvement Programme

Roles and responsibilities

3.16 The new NHS will mean new roles and responsibilities for Health Authorities, NHS Trusts and the Department of Health. Primary Care Groups will also be developed across the country. The facing page sets out the new financing and accountability arrangements compared with those of the internal market.

'leaner bodies with stronger powers'

3.17 Health Authorities will be leaner bodies with stronger powers to improve the health of their residents and oversee the effectiveness of the NHS locally. Over time, they will relinquish direct commissioning functions to Primary Care Groups. Working with local authorities, NHS Trusts and Primary Care Groups, they will take the lead in drawing up three-year Health Improvement Programmes which will provide the framework within which all local NHS bodies will operate. These will be backed by a new duty of partnership. Health Authorities will allocate funds to Primary Care Groups on an equitable basis, and hold them to account. Links with social services will be strengthened. Fewer Health Authorities covering larger areas will emerge as a product of these changes, flowing from local discussion rather than national edict.

'commissioning services'

3.18 Primary Care Groups comprising all GPs in an area together with community nurses will take responsibility for commissioning services for the local community. This will not affect the independent contractor status of GPs. The new Primary Care Groups will replace existing commissioning and fundholding arrangements. All Primary Care Groups will be accountable to Health Authorities, but will have freedom to make decisions about how they deploy their resources within the framework of the Health Improvement Programme. Over time, Primary Care Groups will have the opportunity to become freestanding Primary Care Trusts.

'providing services for patients'

3.19 NHS Trusts, the bodies that provide patient services in hospitals and in the community, will be party to the local Health Improvement Programme and will agree long term service agreements with Primary Care Groups. These service agreements will generally be organised around a particular care group (such as children) or disease area (such as heart disease) linked to the new National Service Frameworks. In this way, hospital clinicians will be able to make a more significant contribution to service planning. National model agreements will be developed. NHS Trusts will have a statutory duty for quality.

3.20 The **Department of Health**, and within it the NHS Executive, will shoulder responsibility for action genuinely needed at a national level. It will integrate health and social services policy to give a national lead which others will be expected to follow locally. It will also work with the clinical professions to develop National Service Frameworks, linked to national action to implement them across the NHS. For the first time, there will be an annual national survey to allow systematic comparisons of the experience of patients and their carers over time, and between different parts of the country. A new NHS Charter will set out new rights and responsibilities for patients. The Secretary of State will have reserve powers to intervene where Health Authorities, Primary Care Groups and NHS Trusts are failing.

'giving a national lead'

3.21 To reflect the new partnership and interdependence at local level, NHS Executive Regional Offices will integrate their performance management functions. The Regional Offices will have new responsibilities for ensuring that Primary Care Groups and Health Authorities work together to make proper arrangements for commissioning specialist health services at a regional level. Regional Chairs will take a stronger role in ensuring local partnerships are developed between the NHS and Local Authorities.

3.22 The following chapters set out the proposals in more detail, showing how they will work and how they will meet the Government's objective of a modern and dependable NHS for patients.

4

Key themes

- *new focus on improving health*
- *new Health Improvement Programmes to shape local healthcare*
- *lead strategic role for local NHS*

Health Authorities
leading and shaping

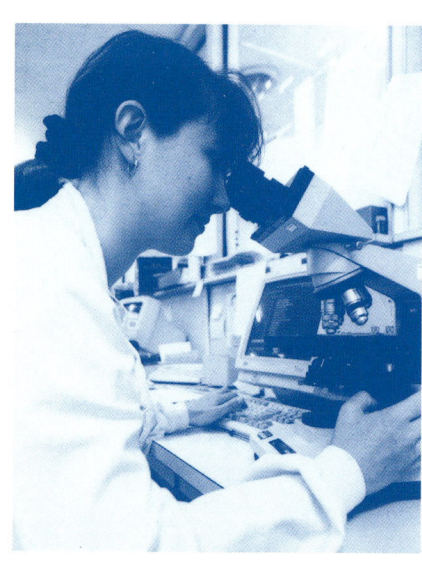

Strategic leadership

4.1 Health Authorities will give strategic leadership on the ground in the new NHS. They will lead the development of local Health Improvement Programmes which will identify the health needs of local people and what needs to be done to meet them. Health Authorities will work closely with NHS Trusts, the new Primary Care Groups, Local Authorities, academic and research interests, voluntary organisations, and the local community in devising this new strategic approach to the planning and delivery of healthcare.

4.2 A stronger, clearer strategic role for Health Authorities will help overcome the fragmentation which characterised the internal market. Now there will be common goals so that each part of the local health service works in concert with one another and in partnership with local government and others. Health Authorities will be freed from unnecessary administrative activities so that they are properly able to lead the local NHS and ensure it delivers. Patients in all parts of the country will feel the benefit through coordinated, high quality and accessible services.

Health Authority functions

4.3 Health Authorities will have a number of key tasks:

- **assessing the health needs** of the local population, drawing on the knowledge of other organisations

- drawing up a strategy for meeting those needs, in the form of a **Health Improvement Programme,** developed in partnership with all the local interests and ensuring delivery of the NHS contribution to it

- deciding on the **range and location of health care services** for the Health Authority's residents, which should flow from, and be part of, the Health Improvement Programme

- determining **local targets and standards** to drive quality and efficiency in the light of national priorities and guidance, and ensuring their delivery

- supporting the **development of Primary Care Groups** so that they can rapidly assume their new responsibilities

- **allocating resources to Primary Care Groups**

- **holding Primary Care Groups to account**.

'improving health and reducing inequalities'

Improving the public's health

4.4 Lead responsibility for improving overall health and reducing health inequalities will be at the heart of the new Health Authority role. Following publication of the Green Paper *Our Healthier Nation*, the Government will introduce legislation to place a new statutory duty on Health Authorities to improve the health of their population.

4.5 But Health Authorities will not work alone. They will act in partnership with Local Authorities and others to identify how local action on social, environmental and economic issues will make most impact on the health of local people. Their public health functions include health surveillance and the control of communicable diseases; assessing health needs; monitoring health outcomes; and evaluating the health impact of local plans and developments. The Chief Medical Officer will recommend shortly how the public health function can be strengthened to support this work.

'they will act in partnership'

4.6 The independent annual report by their Director of Public Health will inform the decisions of both the Health Authority and its partners. It will be the starting point for the Health Improvement Programme.

Health Improvement Programmes

'the first Health Improvement Programmes will be in place by April 1999'

4.7 The Health Improvement Programme will be the local strategy for improving health and healthcare. It will be the means to deliver national targets in each Health Authority area. The Health Authority will have lead responsibility for drawing up the Health Improvement Programme in consultation with NHS Trusts, Primary Care Groups, other primary care professionals such as dentists, opticians and pharmacists, the public, and other partner organisations.

4.8 To give substance to the cooperation necessary to bring about improvements in health there will be a new statutory duty of partnership placed on local NHS bodies to work together for the common good. This will extend to Local Authorities, strengthening the existing requirements under the 1977 NHS Act. The Government intends to place on Local Authorities a duty to promote the economic, social and environmental well being of their areas. This will ensure they have clear powers to develop partnerships with a wide range of other organisations, including NHS bodies, to address the needs of local communities.

4.9 The Health Improvement Programme will cover:

- the most important **health needs** of the local population, and how these are to be met by the NHS and its partner organisations through broader action on public health

- the main **healthcare requirements** of local people, and how local services should be developed to meet them either directly by the NHS, or where appropriate jointly with social services

- the **range, location and investment required in local health services** to meet the needs of local people.

4.10 The initial Health Improvement Programme will cover a three year period. It will be updated progressively, with a part of it reviewed each year. It is envisaged that the first Health Improvement Programmes will be in place by April 1999.

4.11 The Health Authority will monitor the implementation of the Health Improvement Programme by NHS Trusts, Primary Care Groups and others. It will decide on and be required to ensure the delivery of the NHS components. It will therefore have reserve powers to ensure that major investment decisions (such as capital developments or new consultant medical staffing appointments) are consistent with the Health Improvement Programme.

4.12 The Health Authority will also need to ensure the local NHS works in partnership to coordinate plans for the local workforce. Local education consortia should ensure training and education arrangements are in place to provide the skills needed across the hospital and community sectors, primary care and social care. And in order to guarantee that patients have quicker access to local services, the Health Authority will coordinate information and information technology plans across primary care, community health services and secondary care.

> **Local Education Consortia**
>
> Consortia bring together representatives from NHS Trusts and Health Authorities to assess the workforce and development requirements of local healthcare services. They provide a forum to ensure workforce planning reflects local service needs.

4.13 Health Authorities will work more closely with local social services and other partners on planning care for patients. At present, the quality of cooperation varies considerably. Inevitably, the consequence is unfairness between different parts of the country.

4.14 In the future, patients with continuing health and social care needs will get access to more integrated services through the joint investment plans for continuing and community care services which all Health Authorities are being asked to produce with partner agencies. The Government will also be exploring the scope for even closer working between health and social services through, for example, pooling of budgets. The benefits will be particularly felt by patients, such as those with disability or mental health problems, who need the support of both health and social care systems.

'more integrated health and social care services'

Devolving responsibility

4.15 Health Authorities will devolve responsibility for direct commissioning of services to new Primary Care Groups as soon as they are able to take on this task. Such an approach provides a 'third way' between stifling top-down command and control on the one hand, and a random and wasteful grass roots free-for-all on the other. This 'third way' builds on the successes that commissioning groups and fundholders have achieved over recent years. It harnesses the strategic abilities of Health Authorities and the innovative energies of primary care commissioners for the benefit of patients.

4.16 Although most commissioning will pass to Primary Care Groups, Health Authorities will need to work together to commission some specialist services - those organised to serve the population of several Health Authorities, such as bone marrow transplants. The detailed arrangements for specialist services commissioning are described in chapter 7.

Setting standards and targets

'targets that are measurable, published and deliver year on year improvement'

4.17 The Health Improvement Programme will need to include the new targets which emerge following consultation on the Green Paper *Our Healthier Nation* as well as the performance framework set out in chapter 8. Health Authorities will need to agree and set targets for Primary Care Groups in discussion with them. In turn, Primary Care Groups will build them into their service agreements with NHS Trusts. These targets will be measurable, published and deliver year on year improvement in local health and healthcare services.

Holding to account

4.18 The Health Improvement Programme will set the framework, within which Primary Care Groups will consider how best to commission and provide services for their local community. Key objectives including the standards and targets agreed with the Health Authority will be expressed in an annual accountability agreement between the Health Authority and Primary Care Group. Progress will be monitored against this and the Health Authority will hold the Primary Care Group to account for carrying out its agreed role effectively. The detailed arrangements are set out in chapter 5. The service agreements which Health Authorities and Primary Care Groups reach with NHS Trusts will be the chief means of holding NHS Trusts to account for service delivery against the Health Improvement Programme. Where there is a disagreement between a Primary Care Trust and NHS Trusts, it will be for the Health Authority to resolve.

Rebuilding public confidence

4.19 The new arrangements need to be transparent so that they command public confidence. The Government expects Health Authorities to play a strong role in communicating with local people and ensuring public involvement in decision making about the local health service. The maxim to which Health Authorities will work is simple - the NHS, as a public service for local communities, should be both responsive and accountable. Some Health Authorities have been successful in developing new approaches to reflect this maxim. The Government will seek to build on what has worked to ensure this applies everywhere. Health Action Zones will offer opportunities to explore new ways of involving local people. In the meantime, Health Authorities will need to:

- involve the public in developing the Health Improvement Programme

- ensure that Primary Care Groups have effective arrangements for public involvement

- publish agreed strategies, targets and details of progress against them

- participate in a new national survey of patient and user experience (detailed in chapter 8).

4.20 The Government will also take action to rebuild public confidence in the NHS. A new NHS Charter will replace the more limited Patient's Charter. The Government wants a strong public voice in health and healthcare decision-making, recognising the important part played by Community Health Councils in providing information and advice, and in representing the patient's interest. The Government attaches particular importance to strengthening public confidence in the way major changes in local services are planned. We will explore new ways of securing informed public and expert involvement in such decisions. For the first time there will be a clear set of principles for decision-making and criteria for ensuring that due process is observed.

Health Action Zones

A new initiative to bring together organisations within and beyond the NHS to develop and implement a locally agreed strategy for improving the health of local people. Up to 10 zones, generally covering an area of at least Health Authority size, will be selected to go live from April 1998.

'communicating with local people and ensuring public involvement'

The new NHS Charter

The new NHS Charter will tell people about the standards of treatment and care they can expect of the NHS. It will also explain patients' responsibilities.

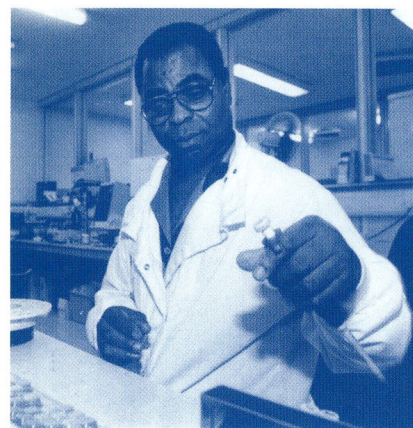

Making it happen

4.21 To support and equip Health Authorities for their significant new role, the Government will:

- revise and clarify their formal responsibilities, with new and specific **statutory responsibilities** for improving the health of the population, and for working in partnership with NHS and other local bodies (which will also be reflected in the duties of partner organisations)

- align NHS Trust and Primary Care Groups' responsibilities and lines of accountability with the new Health Authority role, so that they all work within the local Health Improvement Programme. This will include a specific **reserve power** for the Health Authority to ensure that capital investment and new consultant medical staffing decisions do not cut across the strategy set out in the Health Improvement Programme

- provide for **Local Authority Chief Executives** to participate in meetings of the Health Authority. The Government will also consider further with the NHS and local government how partnership arrangements can be further strengthened, drawing on the experience of Health Action Zones

- work with Health Authorities to **streamline their administrative functions**, including the sharing of functions between Authorities, so as to release time, effort and resources for higher priorities. Fewer authorities covering larger areas will emerge as a product of these changes. Local decision rather than national edict will determine the future Health Authority map.

'fewer authorities covering larger areas'

Ensuring progress

4.22 It will be crucial that Health Authorities make a success of their new role. The NHS Executive will monitor their performance closely, supporting and rewarding good progress, and taking prompt action where necessary to address weaknesses. This will be achieved in three ways:

- firstly, without compromising the principle of allocating resources on the basis of need, Health Authorities which demonstrate most progress against the targets and objectives agreed with the NHS Executive will be eligible for modest extra non-recurrent funding for local projects which support their Health Improvement Programme

- secondly, particular emphasis will be put on benchmarking and on the sharing of good practice

- thirdly, where there are poorly performing authorities, Regional Offices will monitor progress more closely, offer targeted management support, and ultimately will be able to intervene directly to strengthen existing management.

'rewarding success'

Milestones

The initial steps will be:

1998

- prepare the way for development of Primary Care Groups
- first national survey of patient and user experience
- establishment of Health Action Zones
- prepare Health Improvement Programmes

1999

- (subject to legislation) introduction of Health Authorities' new statutory duties
- support for Primary Care Groups in their first year
- the first Health Improvement Programmes begin

5 Key themes

- *development of primary and community health care*
- *family doctors and community nurses in the lead*
- *a spectrum of opportunities beyond fundholding*

Primary Care Groups
going with the grain

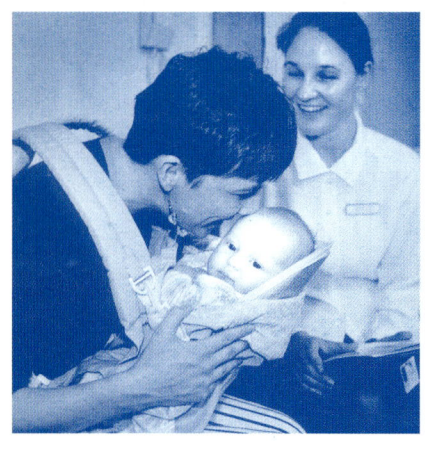

The first line of support and care

5.1 The family doctor or community nurse is often the first port of call for patients when they need health advice or treatment. Primary care professionals are also the way into the rest of the NHS for most patients. They understand patients' needs and they deliver most local services. That is why they will be in the driving seat in shaping local health services in the future. New Primary Care Groups will be established in all parts of the country to commission services for local patients. They will have control over resources but will have to account for how they have used them in improving efficiency and quality. They do not affect GPs' independent contractor status.

'Primary Care Groups will grow out of the range of commissioning models that have developed in recent years'

5.2 The new role envisaged for GPs and community nurses will build on some of the most successful recent developments in primary care. These professionals have seized opportunities to extend their role in recent years. Practice nurses are taking on new disease management roles while community pharmacists are increasingly a source of advice for both GPs and patients. GPs have been developing new services within their surgeries. Health visitors, school nurses, and district nurses have enhanced the delivery of care in homes, schools and the community.

5.3 Community health services have been able to take account of the special health needs of black and minority ethnic patients. They have also been able to help people not in regular contact with other parts of the health services, such as homeless people. Community health staff, such as midwives, can also draw attention to the wider health needs of the community, where the real solution may lie in action on education, housing, transport or reducing air pollution.

Going with the grain

5.4 Extended roles in providing primary and community healthcare have been matched by greater influence in shaping hospital services. Multifunds, locality commissioning groups, individual fundholders, and total purchasing projects all have helped lead the way. Each has undoubtedly brought benefits to patients. The new GP commissioning pilots will extend the range of opportunities. The Government's plans go with the grain of these developments.

5.5 Despite its limitations, many innovative GPs and their fund managers have used the fundholding scheme to sharpen the responsiveness of some hospital services and to extend the range of services available in their own surgeries. But the fundholding scheme has also proved bureaucratic and costly. It has allowed development to take place in a fragmented way, outside a coherent strategic plan. It has artificially separated responsibility for emergency and planned care, and given advantage to some patients at the expense of others.

5.6 So the Government wants to keep what has worked about fundholding, but discard what has not. The potential of primary care commissioning will continue to be developed using mechanisms that evolve far beyond single practice standard fundholding. The argument between fundholding and non-fundholding is yesterday's debate. The time has come to move on, taking the best of both approaches.

5.7 All of the local community should benefit from the best that primary and community health services have to offer. It is at this level - close to patients and the community - that decisions can best be taken on using the resources of the NHS to meet the health and healthcare needs of individual patients.

5.8 The Government therefore intends to establish Primary Care Groups across the country, bringing together GPs and community nurses in each area to work together to improve the health of local people.

Locality commissioning groups

Groups of GPs who work closely with their Health Authority to plan and commission services.

GP fundholding

A GP whose practice manages a budget for its practice staff, certain hospital referrals, drug costs, community nursing services and management costs.

Multifunds

Groups of GP fundholders who agree to pool their budgets and work together.

Total purchasing projects

Total purchasers comprise groups of GPs who together purchase hospital and community health services outside fundholding on behalf of their patients, working closely with their Health Authority. Legal responsibility for these services remains with the relevant Health Authority.

GP commissioning group pilots

Pilot projects preparing to go live from April 1998. Based around groups of fundholding and non-fundholding GPs, will manage a prescribing budget. Will work closely with their local Health Authority to develop health strategies and advise on service developments for local populations.

Community health services

Community health services are provided for people wherever they are, such as in homes, schools, clinics and even on the streets. Examples are health visiting, school nursing, chiropody, speech and language therapy. Services such as district nursing, community psychiatric nursing and physiotherapy can enable people with short or long term illness or disability to be cared for in their own homes.

'child health and rehabilitation services will particularly benefit'

Local Medical Committee

The statutory Local Representative Committee for all GPs in the area covered by a Health Authority. The Health Authority has a statutory duty to consult it on issues including GPs' terms of service, complaints and the investigation of certain matters of professional conduct.

Primary Care Groups will grow out of the range of commissioning models that have developed in recent years but will give a sharper focus to their work. They will have the benefit of strong support from their Health Authority and the freedom to use NHS resources wisely, including savings. With these new opportunities will go the need to account for their actions. They will be subject to clear accountability arrangements and performance standards.

Functions

5.9   The main functions of the new Primary Care Groups reflect the approaches which are already being adopted in many parts of the country. Primary Care Groups will:

- contribute to the Health Authority's **Health Improvement Programme** on health and healthcare, helping to ensure that this reflects the perspective of the local community and the experience of patients

- **promote the health of the local population,** working in partnership with other agencies

- **commission health services** for their populations from the relevant NHS Trusts, within the framework of the Health Improvement Programme, ensuring quality and efficiency

- **monitor performance** against the service agreements they (or initially the Health Authority) have with NHS Trusts

- **develop primary care** by joint working across practices; sharing skills; providing a forum for professional development, audit and peer review; assuring quality and developing the new approach to clinical governance; and influencing the deployment of resources for general practice locally. Local Medical Committees will have a key role in supporting this process

- **better integrate primary and community health services** and work more closely with **social services** on both planning and delivery. Services such as child health or rehabilitation where responsibilities have been split within the health service and where liaison with Local Authorities is often poor, will particularly benefit.

Structure

5.10 The precise form of Primary Care Groups will be flexible to reflect local circumstances. In some areas there are already well established GP-led groups of commissioners or fundholders, while in others, community NHS Trusts have taken a lead role. Successful local arrangements will be built upon, not discarded. The approach will be bottom-up and developmental.

'the approach will be bottom-up and developmental'

5.11 There will be a spectrum of opportunities available for local GPs and community nurses. Primary Care Groups will develop over time, learning from existing arrangements and their own experience. None will affect the independent contractor status of GPs. There will be four options for the form that Primary Care Groups take. They will:

i at minimum, support the Health Authority in commissioning care for its population, acting in an advisory capacity

ii take devolved responsibility for managing the budget for healthcare in their area, formally as part of the Health Authority

iii become established as freestanding bodies accountable to the Health Authority for commissioning care

iv become established as freestanding bodies accountable to the Health Authority for commissioning care and with added responsibility for the provision of community health services for their population.

Primary Care Groups

5.12 Primary Care Groups will begin at whatever point on the spectrum is appropriate for them. They will be expected to progress along it so that in time all Primary Care Groups assume fuller responsibilities. Some Primary Care Groups may proceed directly from option ii to option iv.

'Primary Care Trusts running community health services'

5.13 The Government will bring forward legislation to establish a new form of Trust - a Primary Care Trust - for Primary Care Groups which wish to be freestanding (options iii and iv) and are capable of being so. Such Trusts may include community health services from existing NHS Trusts. All or part of an existing community NHS Trust may combine with a Primary Care Trust in order to better integrate services and management support. Annex A sets out further details of how Primary Care Trusts might work. (Elsewhere in this document, the term Primary Care Group is used to cover both Groups and Trusts, unless the context makes it clear that Groups alone are covered).

5.14 The new Trusts will not be expected to take responsibility for specialised mental health or learning disability services. On mental health, where health and social care boundaries are not fixed and where joint work is particularly important, and where an integrated range of services from community to hospital care is required, specialist mental health NHS Trusts are likely to be the best mechanism for coordinating service delivery. Primary Care Trusts will be well placed to develop strong links with such services. In this way, specialist NHS Trusts, Primary Care Trusts and social services will be able to make complementary contributions to delivering the full range of care. Similar considerations apply in the case of specialist learning disability services.

5.15 Whatever functions they take on there will be a common core of requirements for all Primary Care Groups. Each Group will be accountable to the Health Authority and required to:

- be representative of all the GP practices in the Group

- have a governing body which includes community nursing and social services as well as GPs drawn from the area

- take account of social services as well as Health Authority boundaries, to help promote integration in service planning and provision

- abide by the local Health Improvement Programme

- have clear arrangements for public involvement including open meetings

- have efficient and effective arrangements for management and financial accountability.

Local Medical Committees will continue to be consulted on,

and have a key role in, ensuring that general medical services resources are used wisely.

5.16 The intention is that Primary Care Groups should develop around natural communities, but take account also of the benefits of coterminosity with social services. Practices based close to the borders of a Group will be able to choose to join with others in the way which makes best sense locally. Primary Care Groups may typically serve about 100,000 patients. But there will be flexibility to reflect local circumstances and emerging evidence about the effectiveness of different size groupings. Primary Care Groups will generally grow out of existing local groupings, modified as needed to meet the criteria set out above.

Finance

5.17 Each Primary Care Group will have available their population's share of the available resources for hospital and community health services, prescribing and general practice infrastructure. These resources will allow the Group and its members to commission and provide services. Within this single cash limited envelope, the Group will have the opportunity to deploy resources and savings to strengthen local services and ensure that patterns of care best reflect their patients' needs.

'deploying resources and savings to strengthen local services'

5.18 For the first time in the history of the NHS all the primary care professionals, who do the majority of prescribing, treating and referring, will have control over how resources are best used to benefit patients. By cutting through the artificial barriers that have been erected between drug budgets, hospital referral budgets and emergency admission budgets the Government will give real choices about how GPs and community nurses deploy their cash. In this way Primary Care Groups will extend to all patients the benefits, but not the disadvantages, of fundholding. By virtue of their size and financial leverage, they will have far greater ability to shape local services around patients' needs.

Unified Primary Care Group Budgets

- Hospital and Community Health Services
- Prescribing: the cost of drugs prescribed by GP and nurses
- GMS infrastructure: the current 'GMS cash-limited' budget which reimburses GPs for a proportion of the cost of their practice staff premises and computers.

5.19 Groups, rather than individual practices, will reach service agreements with NHS Trusts about the quality and level of care that should be provided in hospitals for their patients. Primary Care Groups will also work with their practices to ensure the best use of resources for their patients. Over time, the Government expects that Groups will extend indicative budgets to individual practices for the full range of services, but no individual element will be artificially capped. It will be open to the Group to agree practice-level incentive arrangements associated with these budgets, approved by the Health Authority, where this helps promote best use of resources. Initially every practice will have a prescribing budget, as most do now.

Management costs

5.20 Primary Care Groups will have their own dedicated management support, but will be expected to share, not duplicate, functions. In particular, they will work closely together and with their Health Authority to share scarce expertise such as public health skills. Where support functions can most cost-effectively be delegated back to Health Authorities, Primary Care Groups will be expected to do so.

5.21 A combined Health Authority and Primary Care Group management cost envelope will be set for each Health Authority area. The Government will support the development of Primary Care Groups in all parts of the country by fairly redistributing, over time, the management costs that have supported GP fundholding as well as those that have supported Health Authorities' direct commissioning role. GP fundholding only covers part of the country and part of local health services, so by cutting the number of commissioning bodies and scrapping both short-term contracts and individual case contracts, the new arrangements will also cut transaction costs and bureaucracy. That will allow management resources to be used more effectively. It will also help all practices to develop the information systems needed for integrated health care.

5.22 Redeployment of the GP Fundholding Practice Fund Management Allowance will provide about £3 per head of population to support the running costs of Primary Care Groups as part of the overall Health Authority/Primary Care Group cost envelope available locally. Further management support costs will be redeployed over time from Health Authorities as Primary Care Groups take on more responsibilities. GPs who take on key responsibilities within Primary Care Groups will have their time appropriately reimbursed from within the Group's management support.

'by cutting the number of commissioning bodies and scrapping both short-term contracts and individual case contracts, the new arrangements will also cut transaction costs and bureaucracy'

5.23 Where a Primary Care Group merges with a Community NHS Trust the management cost envelope will be further adjusted. The Government will require such mergers to bring significant overall savings in management costs as functions, overheads and support services are combined.

Accountability

5.24 Primary Care Groups and Primary Care Trusts will be accountable to Health Authorities for the way in which they discharge their functions, including financial matters. This will ensure that they work within the Health Improvement Programme and that financial discipline and probity are maintained. In addition the Health Authority and the Primary Care Group will agree targets for improving health, health services and value for money. These will be set out in an annual accountability agreement.

'there will be accountability agreements between Primary Care Groups and Health Authorties'

5.25 Before securing increased responsibility, Groups will need to satisfy the Health Authority that they have adequate management arrangements (including designation of an Accountable Officer), risk management plans for their budgets, and a proper range of partner and public involvement.

5.26 No barriers will be placed in the way of Primary Care Groups which are making good progress. But where a Primary Care Group is falling behind its peers Health Authorities will need to support it through closer monitoring, advice and guidance and greater direction. In the rare event that a Primary Care Group got into serious difficulty the Health Authority would have the power to withdraw some or all of the devolved responsibility or require a change in its leadership and management.

'no barriers will be placed in the way of Primary Care Groups which are making good progress'

Commissioning better services

5.27 The arrangements set out above will give Primary Care Groups the responsibility as well as the tools and incentives with which to develop prompt, accessible and responsive services for local people. They will be encouraged to play an active part in community development and improving health in its widest sense. Health visitors and health promotion professionals will have a strong contribution to make in identifying health needs and implementing the programmes that best address them. Other primary care professionals, such as dentists, optometrists and pharmacists, will need to be drawn in to contribute as appropriate to the planning and provision of services. This must be a coming together of equals with each profession recognising the distinctive contribution of the others. Dentists, pharmacists and optometrists also have their own separate and distinct contributions to make to the NHS and the Government will continue its dialogue with them about how they can best develop it.

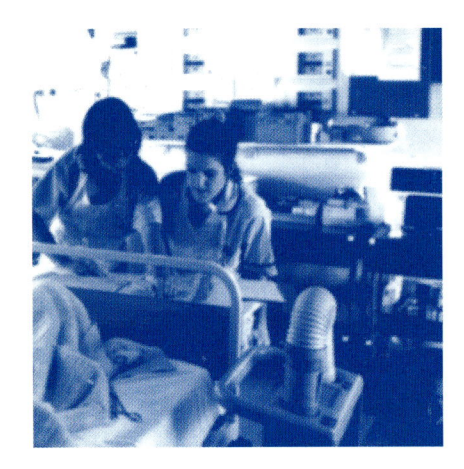

5.28 As part of the commissioning process, Primary Care Groups, Health Authorities and hospital clinicians will agree whether a service should be commissioned for the whole population across the Health Authority, or more locally. Quality standards, service protocols and agreements should be set by direct discussion between clinicians to ensure primary and secondary care services are properly integrated and programmes of care developed to reflect patient needs.

5.29 National Service Frameworks, and guidelines issued by the new National Institute for Clinical Excellence, will help ensure greater local consistency between Health Authorities and Primary Care Groups in the provision of top quality services for major diseases and conditions. In this way devolved commissioning will go hand in hand with greater equity for the most important services, so that two-tierism becomes a thing of the past.

'devolved commissioning will go hand in hand with greater equity'

5.30 Primary Care Groups will be able to make choices about cost-effective patterns of services and will be free to switch resources over time to support them. They will redeploy savings to meet local needs and promote local developments.

Developing primary and community services

5.31 The internal market has over-emphasised the role of primary care as commissioner of hospital services, at the expense of improving the provision of primary care services themselves. Primary Care Groups will set that right. They will be encouraged to use their freedoms to improve primary and community health care for their patients. The independent contractor status of GPs will continue. Working with Health Authorities, Primary Care Groups will be able to use the NHS (Primary Care) Act to pilot local flexibilities in delivering general medical services. Health Authorities will have reserve powers in respect of payments made by Primary Care Groups/Primary Care Trusts to GP practices, for example from general medical services allocations and payments under Section 36 of the Primary Care Act.

5.32 Primary Care Trusts will be able to run community hospitals and other community services. By integrating primary and community healthcare, Primary Care Trusts will provide a focus for improved rehabilitation and recovery services. Too often in the past community hospitals have been sidelined. Their potential contribution to managing the pressures of rising emergency admissions has often been ignored. Patients will be able to use local community hospitals to the full rather than having to travel to more distant acute hospitals. This will be particularly significant in rural areas.

5.33 Primary Care Groups will be expected to help primary care professionals to enhance the quality of their care. There is much on which to build. Clinical audit is now becoming well established in general practice and the NHS Executive is working with the profession to develop indicators to assess the effectiveness of primary care at national and Health Authority level.

5.34 But more is needed. As part of the development of clinical governance in the NHS (discussed in more detail in chapter 6) each Primary Care Group will nominate a senior professional to take the lead on standards generally and on professional development within the Group. To extend this approach through primary care, individual practices will be encouraged to identify lead responsibility on the same basis. Many practices are very small organisations, however, and it will be important to apply the principles of clinical governance sensitively. In order to achieve Primary Care Trust status, Primary Care Groups will need to demonstrate that they have a systematic approach to monitoring and developing clinical standards in practices. This requirement will also be applied to community health services included in the Trust.

Primary Care Act Pilots

Under the NHS (Primary Care) Act 1997, different more flexible ways are being piloted of providing primary care to attune it better to local needs. Pilots will be established from April 1998 to:

- improve the quality, range and accessibility of services
- tackle unmet need for specific groups of people
- improve the recruitment, retention, and develop skills of GPs, nurses and other clinical providers
- establish new organisational models for better providing integrated primary and community healthcare.

'use their freedoms to improve primary and community care'

Beyond fundholding

5.35 Primary Care Groups build on best of existing practice. They offer an opportunity for innovative GPs and community nurses to spread the benefits of their experience more widely. This will ensure that those who are willing and able to lead can do so in a way which benefits all, without requiring every GP to take on a lead management role.

'Primary Care Groups are where the future lies for GP fundholders'

5.36 Primary Care Groups are where the future lies for GP fundholders. The Government will discuss with those concerned an orderly transition covering:

- future arrangements for services currently funded through the fundholding scheme so that those that are cost-effective, including those in GP practices, can continue to be provided, and spread to others

- arrangements for fundholding staff, currently supported from the Practice Fund Management Allowance, so that those skilled in primary care commissioning are wherever possible retained at the practice, Primary Care Group or Health Authority level

- arrangements for winding up Practice Funds, including how savings can be used for the benefit of patients subject to appropriate value-for-money tests.

5.37 The Government will bring forward legislation to provide for the move from GP fundholding to Primary Care Groups and to create the new Primary Care Trusts. Subject to the availability of Parliamentary time for the necessary legislation, Primary Care Groups will succeed fundholding from April 1999. In the meantime, there will be no new admissions to the fundholding scheme.

5.38 In parallel the NHS Executive will:

- explore with all interested parties what can be learned from existing commissioning models, drawing on the extensive programme of research and evaluation currently underway

- ensure Health Authorities work with primary care and community health services locally to develop Primary Care Groups, build on existing local initiatives, and devolve responsibility as new Groups demonstrate the capacity to take it.

Milestones

The development of Primary Care Groups will be evolutionary, building on existing models and the convergence which is already apparent.

1998

- GP Commissioning Group pilots begin
- early action will concentrate on the transition to the new Primary Care Groups

1999

- new Primary Care Groups in place
- GP fundholders, Total Purchasing Projects, multifunds, and locality commissioning GPs will move on to Primary Care Groups and, subject to legislation, the fundholding scheme will be wound up
- Primary Care Groups will take on additional responsibilities at a pace to be agreed locally.

6

Key themes

- *new role helping plan local health services*
- *responsible for operational management*
- *new statutory duties for quality and partnership*
- *new emphasis on staff involvement*

NHS Trusts
partnership and performance

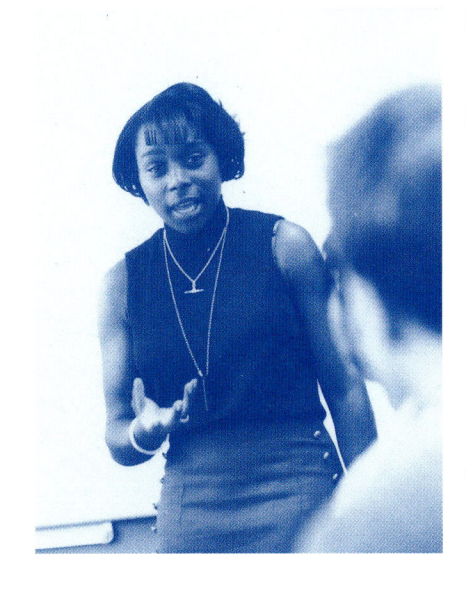

A new direction

6.1 NHS Trusts provide hospital and community health care for millions of patients. They employ the vast majority of NHS staff. Their expenditure accounts for some 72% of the total NHS budget. In partnership with local universities and other research bodies, many NHS Trusts also carry important education and research responsibilities alongside their commitment to patient care. The new NHS will give them a new focus on patients' needs.

6.2 By contrast, market-style incentives drove NHS Trusts to compete to expand their 'business' irrespective of whether this reflected local NHS priorities. Their role was further distorted by the almost exclusive emphasis on their statutory financial duties. The potential contribution of NHS Trusts to both national and local health strategies was undermined.

'clear incentives available to help NHS Trusts succeed'

6.3 Many NHS Trusts tried to overcome the limitations of the market but most found themselves driven by these inappropriate incentives. The proposals in this White Paper will free NHS Trusts to use their managerial and clinical expertise to concentrate on providing improved services for patients. There will be clear incentives available to help NHS Trusts succeed. They will be backed by a tough approach to performance management to drive improvements in quality and efficiency.

6.4 In the new NHS:

- in place of competition, NHS Trusts will as a matter of right **participate in strategy and planning** by helping shape the local Health Improvement Programme

- there will be new **standards for quality and efficiency explicit in local agreements** between Health Authorities, Primary Care Groups and NHS Trusts alongside new measures of efficiency

- **doctors, nurses, and other senior professionals will be much more closely involved** in designing service agreements with commissioners, and in aligning NHS Trust financial priorities with clinical priorities

- **clinical governance** arrangements will be developed in every NHS Trust to guarantee an emphasis on quality

- NHS Trusts will be able to share and **reinvest efficiency gains** to improve services in a way consistent with the local Health Improvement Programme

- **public confidence will be rebuilt** through openness, improved governance and public commitment to the values and aims of the NHS.

'retain full responsibility for operational management'

6.5 These changes will enable NHS Trusts to retain full local responsibility for operational management so that they can make best use of resources for patient care. They will do so within a local service framework that they themselves have played a significant part in creating. They will be accountable to Health Authorities and Primary Care Groups for the services they deliver, and to the NHS Executive for their statutory duties.

Shaping services

6.6 The Government will establish a new statutory duty for NHS Trusts to work in partnership with other NHS organisations. The duty of partnership will require their participation (alongside Primary Care Groups, universities and Local Authorities) in developing the Health Improvement Programme under the leadership of the Health Authority. In turn, the Health Improvement Programme will set the framework for the services NHS Trusts provide and the detailed agreements they make with Primary Care Groups.

'statutory duty for NHS Trusts to work in partnership'

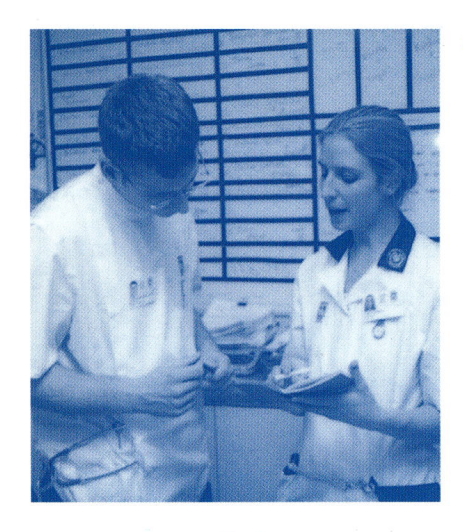

'twin guarantee of consistency and responsiveness'

6.7 Partnership will be dependent on sharing of information with other NHS organisations. The days of the NHS Trust acting alone without regard for others are over. As well as information on progress against service agreements, NHS Trusts will be required to make available their annual operating plans and regular reports on progress against them to local Health Authorities and Primary Care Groups. Key strategic investment decisions, for example in capital, equipment, or in a new consultant post, will need to be consistent with the local Health Improvement Programme.

Focusing on quality

6.8 There will be a new focus on quality in NHS Trusts, so that patients get the twin guarantee of consistency and responsiveness from their local health services. Quality standards will be central to the new local service agreements between Health Authorities, Primary Care Groups and NHS Trusts. New national policies will build on the professional traditions of standard-setting and self-regulation and the good practice which already exists in so many parts of the NHS.

6.9 The Government will establish best practice through the national policies set out in chapter 7. It will strengthen continuing professional development. It will introduce a system of 'clinical governance' in NHS Trusts to guarantee quality.

6.10 In an NHS based on partnership it will be increasingly important for the staff of NHS Trusts to work efficiently and effectively in teams within and across organisational boundaries. Integrated care for patients will rely on models of training and education that give staff a clear understanding of how their own roles fit with those of others within both the health and social care professions. The Government will work with the professions to reach a shared understanding of the principles that should underpin effective continuing professional development and the respective roles of the state, the professions and individual practitioners in supporting this activity.

6.11 NHS Trusts will be expected to strengthen the contribution that nursing can make. To support them in this, the Government will be launching a national consultation on a strategy for nursing, midwifery and health visiting.

Acute and community nursing

The Government is particularly keen to extend the recent developments in the roles of nurses working in acute and community services. Expert nurses are taking on a leadership role, monitoring and educating nurses and other staff, managing care, developing nurse-led clinics and district-wide services. They work across organisational and professional boundaries ensuring continuity and integration of care. The Government is committed to encouraging and supporting the development of nursing practice in these ways.

Clinical governance

6.12 Professional and statutory bodies have a vital role in setting and promoting standards, but shifting the focus towards quality will also require practitioners to accept responsibility for developing and maintaining standards within their local NHS organisations. For this reason the Government will require every NHS Trust to embrace the concept of 'clinical governance' so that quality is at the core, both of their responsibilities as organisations and of each of their staff as individual professionals.

6.13 This new approach to quality will be explicitly reflected in the responsibilities and management of NHS Trusts. Under the internal market, NHS Trusts' principal statutory duties were financial. The Government will bring forward legislation to give them a new duty for the quality of care. Under these arrangements, Chief Executives will carry ultimate responsibility for assuring the quality of the services provided by their NHS Trust, just as they are already accountable for the proper use of resources.

6.14 Chief Executives will be expected to ensure there are appropriate local arrangements to give them and the NHS Trust board firm assurances that their responsibilities for quality are being met. This might be through the creation of a Board Sub-Committee, led by a named senior consultant, nurse, or other clinical professional, with responsibility for ensuring the internal clinical governance of the organisation.

6.15 These arrangements should build on and strengthen the existing systems of professional self-regulation and the principles of corporate governance, but offer a framework for extending this more systematically into the local clinical community. It is important that these arrangements engage professionals at ward and clinical level. NHS Trust boards will expect to receive monthly reports on quality, in the same way as they now receive financial reports, and to publish an annual report on what they are doing to assure quality. Quality will quite literally be on the agenda of every NHS Trust board.

A quality organisation will ensure that:

- quality improvement processes (eg clinical audit) are in place and integrated with the quality programme for the organisation as a whole

- leadership skills are developed at clinical team level

- evidence-based practice is in day-to-day use with the infrastructure to support it

- good practice, ideas and innovations (which have been evaluated) are systematically disseminated within and outside the organisation

- clinical risk reduction programmes of a high standard are in place

- adverse events are detected, and openly investigated; and the lessons learned promptly applied

- lessons for clinical practice are systematically learned from complaints made by patients

- problems of poor clinical performance are recognised at an early stage and dealt with to prevent harm to patients

- all professional development programmes reflect the principles of clinical governance

- the quality of data collected to monitor clinical care is itself of a high standard.

Driving performance

'a new duty for the quality of care'

6.16 In the new NHS, the performance of NHS Trusts will be assessed against new broad-based measures reflecting the wider goals of improving health and healthcare outcomes, the quality and effectiveness of service, efficiency and access. Performance will be judged by greater use of comparative information. Details are contained in chapter 8.

6.17 NHS Trusts and their clinical teams will be held to account on this new basis through their service agreements with Health Authorities and increasingly Primary Care Groups. These will stipulate quality measures so that patient services meet demanding targets for responsiveness. They will be longer-term agreements often covering a minimum of three years (see chapter 9 for more details) rather than the current annual contracts. The longer-term agreements will provide NHS Trusts with incentives to ensure appropriate levels of service usage, replacing incentives simply to increase hospital admissions, whether they were required or not.

6.18 With longer-term agreements will come greater stability for NHS Trusts so that they can confidently plan ahead for changes and improvements in the services they provide. The best NHS Trusts of the future will play their full part in shaping and delivering quality healthcare for the local community, confident of the distinctive contribution they have to make, but respecting the contribution of others, and where appropriate willing to see services move to other organisations.

'when performance is not up to scratch in NHS Trusts there will be rapid investigation and, when necessary, intervention'

6.19 NHS Trusts will be accountable to the relevant NHS Executive Regional Office for fulfilling their statutory duties and for their effective operation as public bodies. The effect of their new statutory duties will be to broaden their accountability which until now has rested largely on financial performance. In future they will need also to be able to demonstrate that they have the necessary systems in place to assure quality, and are working in partnership within the framework of the Health Improvement Programme.

6.20 In the new NHS, when performance is not up to scratch in NHS Trusts there will be rapid investigation and, where necessary, intervention. This will take five forms:

- firstly, Health Authorities will be able to call in the NHS Executive Regional Offices when it appears that an NHS Trust is failing to deliver against the Health Improvement Programme

- secondly, NHS Executive Regional Offices will be able to investigate if there is a question over compliance with their statutory duties

- thirdly, the Commission for Health Improvement could be called in to investigate and report on a problem

- fourthly, Primary Care Groups will be able to signal a change to their local service agreements, where NHS Trusts are failing to deliver

- fifthly, the Secretary of the State could remove the NHS Trust Board.

'efficiency will be enhanced... clinician to clinician partnership'

Promoting efficiency

6.21 Efficiency will be enhanced through incentives at both NHS Trust and clinical team level. Many NHS Trusts already devolve budgetary responsibility to clinical teams and involve senior professionals from them directly in the management of the NHS Trust. All NHS Trusts should be developing these approaches. Increasingly, clinical teams will develop and agree the new longer term service agreements with Primary Care Groups. Clinician to clinician partnership will focus service agreements on securing genuine health gain. The efficiency incentives that come with budgetary responsibility will be reinforced by longer term service agreements that allow a share of any savings made to be redeployed by the clinical teams, in a way consistent with the NHS Trust's priorities and the local Health Improvement Programme.

'longer-term service agreements to allow any savings to be redeployed'

6.22 Partnerships between secondary and primary care clinicians and with social services will provide the necessary basis for the establishment of 'programmes of care', which will allow planning and resource management across organisational boundaries.

6.23 The requirement for benchmarking will encourage rigorous scrutiny of NHS Trusts' costs and performance. All NHS Trusts will in future publish the costs of the treatments they offer, so that inefficient performance can be identified and tackled. Further details are in chapter 9. The new performance framework described in chapter 8 will ensure over time that data are available locally on the areas that matter most to patients as a basis for planning change and measuring progress.

Programmes of care

An example is services for patients with diabetes covering support both in primary care and from specialist hospital services, planned as an integrated whole to meet patients' needs over time.

'less bureaucracy and administration, but more good management'

6.24 Efficiency will also be achieved by bearing down on bureaucracy. The abolition of the internal market will mean a significant reduction in transaction costs, the end of extra-contractual referrals and progressive improvements in efficiency. Together these changes will make it possible to redeploy £1 billion into patient care over the lifetime of this Parliament.

6.25 The move from the market will allow NHS Trust managers to refocus their efforts on the core purposes of the NHS. They will have a critical role in leading the developments set out in this White Paper. The Government wants to see less bureaucracy and administration, but more good management. They are quite different things.

6.26 The Government certainly does not want to see reorganisation for the sake of it. Given the intended integration of primary and community health services, merging community with acute NHS Trusts will not generally be encouraged. Nor will amalgamation of smaller community NHS Trusts be encouraged if this inhibits closer working with local primary care teams. Other mergers arising from local decisions will be considered on their merits, on the basis of demonstrable benefits in health and healthcare, and savings in administration.

Involving staff

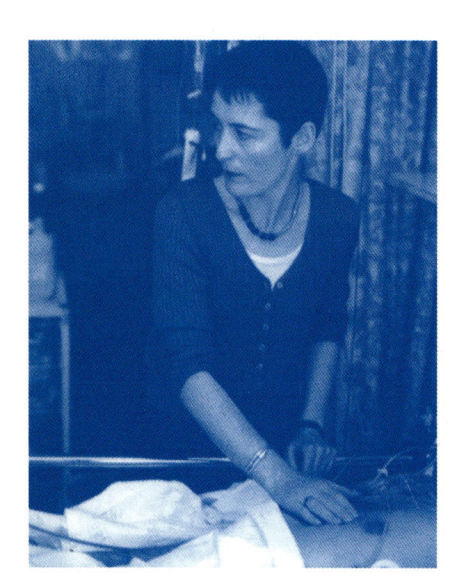

6.27 To succeed in the NHS of the future, NHS Trusts will need to develop and involve their staff. In the past this has not been a high priority. In the new NHS it is - for one simple reason. The health service relies on the commitment and motivation of its staff. That is why there will be a new approach to better valuing staff and NHS Trusts will spearhead it.

6.28 NHS Trusts will retain their role as local employers within the NHS. In a *national* health service, the current mix of national and local contracts is divisive and costly. The Government's objective for the longer term is therefore to see staff receive national pay, if this can be matched by meaningful local flexibility, since current national terms of service for a multitude of staff groups are regarded as inequitable and inflexible. Exploratory discussions on these issues are already under way with staff organisations and NHS employers.

6.29 Pay is but one factor in how staff are rewarded. The Government will work with the NHS to give a higher priority to human resource development. We are currently consulting on a new direction for human resources to encompass action on all issues that affect the quality of the working lives of NHS staff. It will particularly emphasise the need to bring equality and development issues into the mainstream work of the NHS.

'a higher priority to human resource development'

6.30 The NHS Executive has already asked NHS Trusts to tackle a range of immediate human resource priorities. These include measures to promote health at work, through strategies to minimise accidents, avoid violence, and address stress; to recognise and deal with racism; to develop flexible, family-friendly employment policies; to ensure junior doctors have reasonable standards of food and accommodation when on call; and to make sure that staff can speak out when necessary, without victimisation.

'flexible, family-friendly, employment policies'

6.31 Involving staff in service developments and planning change, with open communication and collaboration, is the best way for the NHS to improve patient care. In the future, NHS Trusts will be expected to be open with and involve their own staff. Open communication, including early discussion of any changes, is part of good management, and all staff should have greater opportunities to contribute their ideas for service improvement. All NHS Trusts should work imaginatively through staff consultative committees and other local arrangements to improve dialogue about decisions affecting local health services.

6.32 Nationally, the Government will establish a Taskforce on improving the involvement of frontline staff in shaping new patterns of healthcare. This will identify and explore new approaches and examples of good practice within the NHS and elsewhere. The Taskforce will involve NHS staff, unions, professional bodies, employers and others. It will provide targeted support and advice, and help developing networks of NHS Trusts interested in taking forward this approach locally. It will not duplicate established NHS industrial relations processes.

'taskforce on improving the involvement of frontline staff'

6.33 There will be two further changes:

- NHS Trust Boards will be required to review regularly whether they are doing enough to involve staff

- in their annual reports, NHS Trusts will outline their local policy on staff involvement and include the outcome of any negotiations or local initiatives which have been undertaken throughout the year.

'greater involvement of clinical professionals'

6.34 The best NHS Trusts are already promoting greater involvement of clinical professionals in their management. In the future it will be essential for the professional and managerial environment in every NHS Trust to support clinical behaviour which maximises the quality of care patients receive, minimises waste in the way care is offered and makes best use of the skills of nurses, consultants, junior doctors, and other clinical professionals and support staff.

6.35 It will be important for the right information to be made available to clinicians and for high professional standards to be set and monitored. Equally that the substantial sums invested in education and training support the service objectives of the NHS, and that contractual obligations and incentives support quality, efficiency and effectiveness.

Regional Education Development Groups

Regional Education and Development Groups bring together the key human resources interests at regional level. They advise Regional Offices on the coherence of consortia workforce plans and on the strategic direction of education and training, and ensure that education responds to service needs and developments.

6.36 The NHS Executive and its Regional Offices will provide support through a specific development programme to support the changes set out in this White Paper. The Regional Education Development Groups and local Education Consortia will need to ensure that connections are made between personal and organisational development, and that local and national programmes are complementary.

Rebuilding public confidence

6.37 Greater involvement among staff in NHS Trusts will help rebuild public confidence in the NHS. That confidence was badly dented by the sense that the ethos of the internal market was at odds with health service values.

6.38 In the internal market, NHS Trusts were established as independent statutory corporations, owning assets, and with a financial regime modelled on the private sector. In abolishing the internal market, the Government will amend the NHS Trust financial regime to make it more transparent and more suitable for a public service based on partnership. Control of the estate, comprising land and property, will be retained by NHS Trusts, but Health Authorities will be responsible for monitoring its utilisation to ensure consistency with Health Improvement Programmes and locally agreed estates strategies. The Government will take reserve powers to ensure that the estate is managed in ways which are consistent with local strategies and the broader requirements of the NHS.

'the Government will make NHS Trusts more open and accountable'

6.39 In addition, the Government will make NHS Trusts more open and accountable. Already action has been taken to ensure that NHS Trusts hold their meetings in public and that Board membership is more representative of the local community. To buttress these changes, no management information in the future will be classified as 'commercial in confidence' between NHS bodies. Such a classification is simply not appropriate for organisations that are publicly funded and accountable and are expected to operate as trusted partners working together to the common goal of better health and healthcare for local people.

6.40 Finally NHS Trusts will be expected to publish annually details of their performance, explicitly reflecting the six new dimensions of performance outlined in chapter 8. From 1999 - 2000, their annual accounts will have to include a statement detailing their clinical governance arrangements, drawing on the approach above.

'no management information to be "commercial in confidence" between NHS bodies'

Making it happen

6.41 The new arrangements go with the grain of what NHS Trusts and their staff want. The expectations laid on NHS Trusts are challenging, requiring good leadership and a positive approach to partnership. The commitment of all concerned will be needed to develop their new role as full participants in the local health service. Formal changes in duties will be introduced through legislation but the new approach to partnership is already developing (for example in the 1998-99 commissioning round) and will continue to grow.

Milestones

1998

- new partnership arrangements will develop, and NHS Trusts will participate in preparation of the first Health Improvement Programmes

- a strategic plan for improving human resource management in the NHS will be published

1999

- (subject to legislation) the new framework of statutory duties will be put in place

- new clinical governance arrangements will be put in place to the same timetable

Key themes

- *national leadership to support local development*
- *new National Institute for Clinical Excellence*
- *new Commission for Health Improvement*

The national dimension
a one-nation NHS

7.1 The White Paper aims to renew the NHS as a one-nation health service offering fairness and consistency to the population as a whole. At the same time, the proposals in the White Paper ensure that the NHS delivers a personal service which is sensitive and responsive to the needs of individual patients. The Department of Health, and within it the NHS Executive, have key roles in helping to achieve an appropriate balance between national consistency and local responsiveness.

7.2 The development of new roles and responsibilities for Health Authorities, Primary Care Groups and NHS Trusts will help the NHS meet these objectives. But it is the job of the Department of Health and the NHS Executive with its Regional Offices to provide leadership and support to enable changes to take place across the NHS. They will give national drive to improved quality and improved performance in all parts of the health service.

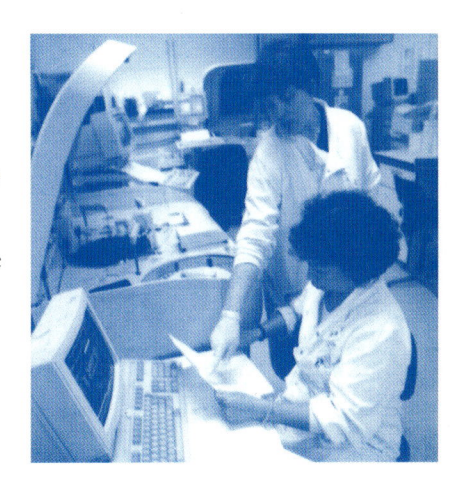

'national drive to improve quality and performance'

7.3 The Department of Health will integrate policy on public health, social care and the NHS so that there is a clear national framework within which similar service development can take place locally. The NHS Executive will develop and implement policy for the NHS. The Government will continue to ensure the costs of the Department of Health and NHS Executive are subject to the same rigour as management costs within the NHS itself. As fewer and larger Health Authorities emerge alongside the development of Primary Care Groups, the role of NHS Executive Regional Offices will need to be kept under review.

Leading on quality

7.4 The NHS Executive and its Regional Offices will be charged with ensuring that quality and responsiveness are instilled at all levels in the NHS. Of course, service quality is essentially determined at local level, through the personal interaction between NHS staff and patients, and the leadership of local management in creating an environment where quality is always to the fore. But there are steps that need to be taken nationally to improve equity and provide a framework for local action.

> 'the Government will spread best practice and drive clinical and cost-effectiveness'

7.5 The Government is determined that the services and treatment that patients receive across the NHS should be based on the best evidence of what does and does not work and what provides best value for money (clinical and cost-effectiveness). At present there are unjustifiable variations in the application of evidence on clinical and cost-effectiveness. All too often in the past, the same problem has been partially solved in different areas. Best practice has not been shared as it should have been. As a result patients have not had fair access to the best the NHS has to offer.

7.6 The Government will spread best practice and drive clinical and cost-effectiveness in a number of ways:

- by ensuring through the **Research and Development Programme** the provision and dissemination of high quality scientific evidence on the cost-effectiveness and quality of care

- by developing a programme of new **evidence-based National Service Frameworks** setting out the patterns and levels of service which should be provided for patients with certain conditions

- by establishing a new **National Institute of Clinical Excellence** which will promote clinical and cost-effectiveness by producing clinical guidelines and audits, for dissemination throughout the NHS

- by establishing a new **Commission for Health Improvement** to support and oversee the quality of clinical governance and of clinical services

- by working with the professions to strengthen the existing systems of **professional self-regulation**

> 'working with the professions to strengthen self-regulation'

Research and Development

7.7 The NHS R&D programme already supports a major programme of research assessing the clinical and cost-effectiveness of health technologies. A new programme of work on service delivery and organisation will look at how care is organised. It will provide research-based evidence about how services can be improved to increase the quality of patient care. In addition, the NHS Executive will take a systematic approach to scanning the horizon for emerging clinical innovations. This will help to set research priorities, to provide information for planning services, and to identify the need for clinical and service guidelines which the new National Institute may be commissioned to develop. The R&D programme will also work to improve access to research findings across the NHS, including the development of a new database.

National Service Frameworks

7.8 The Government will work with the professions and representatives of users and carers to establish clearer, evidence-based **National Service Frameworks** for major care areas and disease groups. That way patients will get greater consistency in the availability and quality of services, right across the NHS. The Government will use them as a way of being clear with patients about what they can expect from the health service.

> **Calman Hine Cancer Report**
>
> The report *A Policy Framework for Commissioning Cancer Services* was commissioned in response to concerns about variations in treatment across the country. It recommended that cancer services should be organised at three levels: primary care; cancer units in local hospitals with multi-disciplinary teams able to treat the commoner cancers; and cancer centres situated in larger hospitals to treat the less common cancers and support cancer units with services such as radiotherapy, not available in smaller hospitals.

7.9 The new approach to developing cancer services in the Calman-Hine Report, and recent action to ensure all centres providing children's intensive care meet agreed national standards, point the direction. In each case, the best evidence of clinical and cost-effectiveness is taken together with the views of users to establish principles for the pattern and level of services required. These then establish a clear set of priorities against which local action can be framed. The NHS Executive, working with the professions and others, will develop a similar approach to other services where national consistency is desirable. There will be an annual programme for the development of such frameworks starting in 1998.

Clinical and cost-effectiveness

7.10 There is a growing body of evidence on which treatments, drugs and other aspects of clinical practice are the most effective and offer

'patients will get greater consistency in the availability and quality of services right across the NHS'

best value. But it is not always easy for frontline doctors and nurses to find the evidence they need. Research results are not readily accessible and it is often difficult for busy health professionals to find their way through the proliferation of emerging guidelines, some of which are of variable quality. To ensure consistent access to beneficial care right across the NHS, the Government believes stronger arrangements are needed to promote clinical and cost effectiveness, both for drugs and other forms of treatment.

National Institute for Clinical Excellence

7.11 A new National Institute for Clinical Excellence will be established to give new coherence and prominence to information about clinical and cost-effectiveness. It will produce and disseminate:

- clinical guidelines based on relevant evidence of clinical and cost-effectiveness

- associated clinical audit methodologies and information on good practice in clinical audit

- in doing so it will bring together work currently undertaken by the many professional organisations in receipt of Department of Health funding for this purpose

- it will work to a programme agreed with and funded from current resources by the Department of Health.

'new coherence and prominence to information about clinical and cost-effectiveness'

7.12 The National Institute's membership will be drawn from the health professions, the NHS, academics, health economists and patient interests. It will need to have access to an appropriate range of skills, including economic and managerial expertise as well as specialist input on specific issues. The Government will consider developing the role and function of the National Institute as it gathers momentum and experience.

Commission for Health Improvement

7.13 To ensure the drive for excellence is instilled throughout the NHS, the Government will create a new **Commission for Health Improvement.** It will complement the introduction of clinical governance arrangements. Past performance on quality has been variable, and the health service has sometimes been slow to detect and act decisively on serious lapses in quality. As a statutory body, at arm's length from Government, the new Commission will offer an independent guarantee that local systems to monitor, assure and improve clinical quality are in place. It will support local development and 'spot-check' the new arrangements. It will also have the capacity to offer targeted support on request to local organisations facing specific clinical problems.

> *'an independent guarantee that local systems to monitor, assure and improve clinical quality are in place'*

7.14 Where local action is not able to resolve serious or persistent problems, the Commission will be able to intervene on the direction of the Secretary of State or by invitation from Primary Care Groups, Health Authorities and NHS Trusts. In these instances, the Commission will both investigate and identify the source of the problem, and work with the organisation on lasting remedies. It will also be able to recommend to the Secretary of State other immediate action. He will have powers to remove NHS Trust Chairs and non-executive directors where there is evidence of systematic failure. The Commission may also undertake an agreed programme of systematic service reviews, following through implementation of the National Service Frameworks and the guidelines developed by the Institute. The Commission will have a membership drawn from the professions, NHS, academic and patient representatives. It will be funded from existing resources.

Professional self-regulation

7.15 Together, these arrangements should ensure that there are stronger systematic measures to monitor, maintain and improve quality. In the rare instances of serious service difficulty, there will now be the capacity for prompt and effective intervention. But the Government will continue to look to individual health professionals to be responsible for the quality of their own clinical practice. Professional self-regulation must remain an essential element in the delivery of quality patient services. It is crucial that the professional standards developed nationally continue to be responsive to changing service needs and to legitimate public expectations. The Government will continue to work with the professions, the regulatory bodies, the NHS and patient representative groups to strengthen the existing systems of professional self-regulation by ensuring that they are open, responsive and publicly accountable.

> *'the capacity for prompt and effective intervention'*

The national dimension

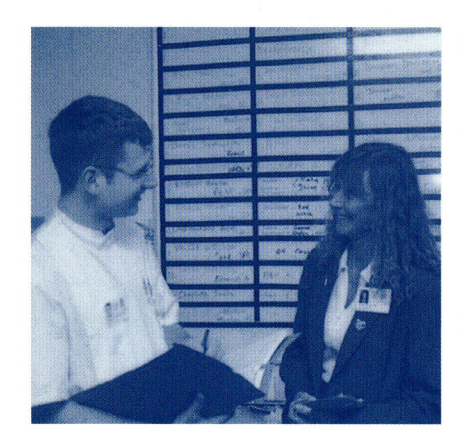

Leading on performance

7.16 The NHS Executive will be responsible for ensuring that the changes in this White Paper are implemented effectively and deliver the improvements that must be made.

7.17 NHS Executive Regional Offices will hold Health Authorities to account for progress in their new strategic leadership role. There will be annual agreements and longer term objectives agreed between the Regional Office and Health Authority on the basis of the local Health Improvement Programme. The Health Authority will be held to account for progress against these.

7.18 Regional Offices will hold NHS Trusts accountable for their new range of statutory duties, with powers to intervene on behalf of the Secretary of State if difficulties - over quality, or over local partnership working within the Health Improvement Programme - cannot be promptly resolved locally.

7.19 To reflect the new partnership and interdependence at local level Regional Offices will integrate their performance management functions. They will also look beyond the roles of individual parts of the NHS to take an overview of the way all parts of the health service in an area are together serving their local population.

7.20 They will look at performance in the round. The new performance framework set out in chapter 8 identifies the range of areas on which the NHS needs to make progress, and sets action in train to measure and manage progress on each of them. This new approach will enable management at all levels to look both at what is being achieved by the NHS as a whole for the local population and to examine the contribution of individual institutions. Regional Offices will drive the new approach to benchmarking, ensuring poor practice is challenged and good practice is identified and spread.

7.21 Looking beyond the NHS, Regional Offices with the Department's Regional Social Services Inspectorate will jointly lead and monitor local action to strengthen partnerships across health and social care and will jointly review progress in areas such as continuing care and mental health. In addition, better integration of policy-making will require closer working relationships between Regional Offices and other parts of Government operating at a regional level.

'Regional Offices will ensure local health services are working together to serve local people'

The national dimension

7.22 The Regional Offices under the direction of the NHS Executive will also give increased priority to supporting and developing the local leaders who will be critical to the new NHS. Regional Offices will participate in the appointment of Health Authority and NHS Trust Chief Executives as well as supporting and monitoring their development.

'supporting and developing local leaders'

Commissioning specialist services

7.23 There is a further new function that will be central to the Regional Office role - providing the means to commission specialist hospital services. The internal market's fragmentation between multiple fundholders and Health Authorities made it difficult to ensure properly coordinated commissioning arrangements for these very specialised services. They are needed for highly complex treatments (such as bone marrow transplants and medium secure psychiatric services) where one centre covers the population of a number of Health Authorities.

7.24 Although Health Authorities have begun to work together voluntarily to plan and fund these services, the results are patchy. A more systematic approach is needed if fair access is to be guaranteed and if clinical staff are to be supported in developing the most suitable and effective care. The Government will therefore introduce new arrangements for planning and commissioning specialist services.

7.25 As a first step, the NHS Executive will discuss with healthcare professionals and managers which services need to be commissioned for populations larger than those of a single Health Authority but below the national level covered by the existing National Specialist Commissioning Advisory Group and the High Secure Psychiatric Services Commissioning Board.

'a more systematic approach to guarantee fair access'

7.26 Regional Offices will be accountable for ensuring that effective arrangements for commissioning these services are established in each Region. There are a number of ways in which such arrangements have been and could be established, but the principles are clear. Health Authorities and Primary Care Groups will be required to participate in them. The arrangements should be capable of commanding the confidence of the clinical units concerned, while being clearly accountable to the Health Authorities and Primary Care Groups on whose behalf they will be commissioning services.

The national dimension

> *'clear quality control and assurance'*

Regional Offices will need to ensure that clear quality control and assurance mechanisms are in place, while bureaucracy is minimised.

7.27 The NHS Executive will discuss with the professions, Health Authorities and NHS Trusts the best way of achieving these aims, drawing on the recent recommendations of the Audit Commission. Regional Offices will ensure that proper arrangements are in place so as effectively to commission specialist services from 1 April 1999.

7.28 Regional Offices have a further role - to make sure breast cancer and cervical cancer screening programmes are subject to proper mechanisms of quality assurance.

Rebuilding public confidence

7.29 The NHS Executive will support the range of initiatives set out in this White Paper on greater involvement for the public, patients and carers. Regional Chairs will promote regional and local partnerships with the community, including stronger working links between the NHS and local government. They will work with local NHS Trust and Health Authority Chairs and non-executive directors, to ensure they are ready to lead their organisations to build the new NHS of the future. At the same time the NHS Executive will involve users and carers in its own work programme.

> *'the NHS Executive will involve users and carers in its own work programme'*

Milestones

1998
- new Information Management and Technology Strategy for the NHS published
- consultation document on quality issues includes proposals for new National Institute for Clinical Excellence, and Commission for Health Improvement
- discussions with the professions, regulatory bodies, NHS and patient representative groups to strengthen professional self-regulation

1999
- subject to legislation, Institute and Commission established
- new arrangements for commissioning specialist services

8

Key themes

- *new measures of NHS performance*
- *action to tackle unacceptable service variations*
- *new national survey of patient experience*

Measuring progress
better every year

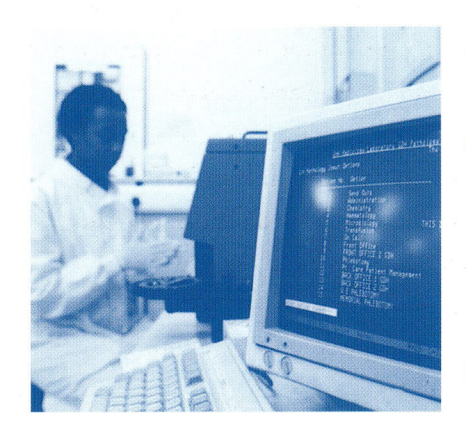

Measuring what counts

8.1 The changes in this White Paper equip Health Authorities, Primary Care Groups and NHS Trusts to discharge their new roles and responsibilities. There are clear incentives and sanctions to help them improve performance.

8.2 There must be improvements in quality and efficiency. Improvements in speed of access to care. Improvements in health, tackling past inequalities. The Government requires the new NHS to make progress on all these fronts. A new national performance framework, measuring how local services are progressing against their targets, will help shape NHS services to meet the challenge.

'the way performance is measured and targets are set drives the way the NHS performs'

8.3 Under the NHS internal market, performance was driven by what could readily be measured: the financial bottom line and the numbers of 'finished consultant episodes'. The Purchaser Efficiency Index, by being based on these measures, failed to reflect the breadth of what patients expect of the service, and of what staff want to provide. It has had a perverse impact on NHS performance. NHS Trusts, for example, were rewarded for hospitalising patients even where more appropriate treatments may have been given in the community. The experience of the internal market has shown that the way performance is measured and targets are set drives the way the NHS performs. Too narrow a focus or the wrong choice of measures distort priorities within the health service.

Measuring progress

The new framework

'there will no longer be a narrow obsession with counting activity for the sake of it'

8.4 The new national performance framework will focus on six areas of performance, selected to capture what really counts for patients and for staff. There will no longer be a narrow obsession with counting activity for the sake of it. Use of the new framework will make it clear to the public and to all those working in the NHS where performance needs to improve. The success of the new NHS will be judged on whether it makes improvements across all areas of the new framework.

8.5 The new framework will demonstrate progress on the overall goals of the NHS, on the key steps the NHS must take to deliver those goals, and on the outcomes it is achieving. It will have six dimensions:

i **Health improvement**
To reflect the overall aim of improving the general health of the population, which is influenced by many factors, reaching well beyond the NHS.

For example, changes in rates of premature death, reflecting social and economic factors as well as healthcare.

ii **Fair access**
To recognise that the NHS contribution must begin by offering fair access to health services in relation to people's needs, irrespective of geography, class, ethnicity, age or sex.

For example, ensuring that black and minority ethnic groups are not disadvantaged in terms of access to services.

iii **Effective delivery of appropriate healthcare**
To recognise that fair access must be to care that is effective, appropriate and timely, and complies with agreed standards.

For example, increasing provision of treatments proven to bring benefit such as hip replacements, provision of rehabilitation at the point when it can offer most benefit, sustained delivery of health and social care to those with long-term needs, and reducing inappropriate treatments.

iv **Efficiency**
The way in which the NHS uses its resources to achieve value for money.

How the new performance framework might work for coronary heart disease

- variations in death rates and risk factors (such as smoking, diet and exercise) across different population groups, for example women or ethnic minorities **(health improvement)**

- ensuring that services are provided fairly, in relation to need, for effective treatments such as cholesterol-lowering therapy or angioplasty **(fair access)**

- reducing the time it takes for heart attack patients to receive clot-busting drugs **(effective healthcare delivery)**

- where appropriate, reducing the length of stay in intensive care after coronary heart surgery; or variations in the cost of coronary artery bypass surgery **(efficiency)**

- increasing patient satisfaction with the management of their care for coronary heart disease, including shorter waiting times for heart operations **(patient/carer experience)**

- success in increasing survival rates and reducing illnesses (such as angina or second heart attacks) in patients treated for known coronary heart disease **(health outcomes of NHS care)**

For example, length of hospital stay; day surgery rates; unit costs; labour productivity; management overhead; capital productivity.

The NHS will be able to assess the impact it has made through offering **fair access** to **effective** care, **efficiently** delivered, by two further measures:

v Patient/carer experience
Through measuring the way in which patients and carers view the quality of the treatment and care that they receive, ensuring the NHS is sensitive to individual needs.

New national patient survey, new NHS Charter.

vi Health outcomes of NHS care
And finally, through assessing the direct contribution of NHS care to improvements in overall health, completing the circle back to the overarching goal of improved health.

For example, trends in infectious diseases for which immunisation programmes are available.

Health Authority Cervical Screening Rates in Women Aged 25-64 at March 1996

Differences from average HA coverage of 85%

8.6 The new framework will allow a more rounded assessment of NHS performance. For this reason, without letting up on the drive for genuine efficiency, the Government will be replacing the Purchaser Efficiency Index from 1 April 1999 with measures based on the new broader performance framework. This approach represents a huge break with the past.

8.7 The public expects a one-nation NHS, with consistent standards and services, wherever they live. The single-minded focus on the old market-driven measures of performance disguised the wide variations that exist in the level and quality of services provided. The new performance framework will encourage greater benchmarking of performance in different areas, and the publication of comparative information will allow people to compare performance and share best practice. Coupled with the new National Service Frameworks, the Government will use these measures for a systematic drive to challenge and reduce unacceptable variations in all aspects of performance across the NHS.

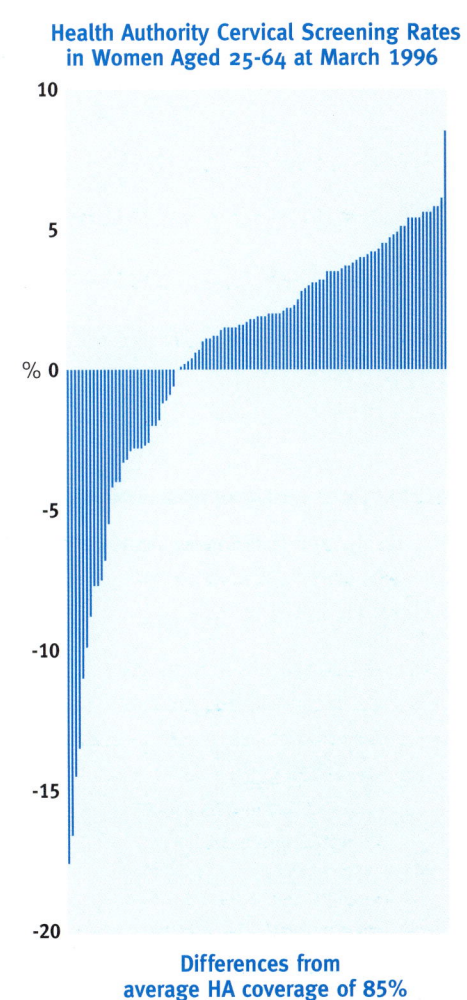

'greater benchmarking of performance'

Measuring progress

8.8 The new framework will be used to chart progress for the population of a Health Authority or Primary Care Group, or to focus on the performance of a particular organisation. It can also be used to examine progress in tackling a particular health problem, and to take a wider look at the delivery of care at the interface between health and social services.

'a new NHS charter'

8.9 As part of the new framework, the Government will take special steps to ensure the experience of users and carers is central to the work of the NHS. The current Patient's Charter was introduced without adequate consultation, and concentrated too much on narrow measures of process. A new NHS Charter will therefore be developed in partnership with NHS users and carers and the staff of the service. It will place greater emphasis on the outcomes of treatment and care. It will focus on things that really matter.

'the health service will measure itself against the aspirations and experience of its users'

8.10 But more is needed. The NHS does not have systematic information about what patients feel about the care it offers. The Government will therefore introduce a new national survey of patient and user experience. It will be carried out annually, at Health Authority level, and the results will be published both locally and nationally. This means that for the first time in the history of the NHS there will be systematic evidence to enable the health service to measure itself against the aspirations and experience of its users, to compare performance across the country and to look at trends over time. The survey will give patients and their carers a voice in shaping the modern and dependable NHS. The first survey will take place in 1998.

Next Steps

'first national survey will take place in 1998'

8.11 The Government will shortly be publishing a consultation document on the details of the new performance framework and proposals for taking it forward. Subject to the results of the consultation, the NHS Executive will develop new high level indicators as a basis for tracking the six areas of performance through all aspects of the way the new NHS is managed. The Green Paper will develop further targets on improving the nation's health.

8.12 Targets for progress against the six parts of the performance framework will be built into:

- the performance agreements between the NHS Executive's Regional Offices and Health Authorities

- local Health Improvement Programmes

- accountability agreements between Primary Care Groups and Health Authorities

- the long term agreements between the new Primary Care Groups and NHS Trusts

- and the way in which the NHS accounts to the public for its performance.

Milestones

1998

- consultation document on the detail of the new performance framework

- the NHS Executive will roadtest a high level indicator, set with Health Authorities, to begin measuring progress on the new basis

- the first national survey of patient and user experience

1999

- end of Purchaser Efficiency Index and introduction of new performance framework

- the NHS will begin to report performance on this new basis, nationally and locally

9

Key themes

- *promoting quality and efficiency*
- *stable funding*
- *fair budgets*
- *£1 billion from bureaucracy*

How the money will flow
from red tape to patient care

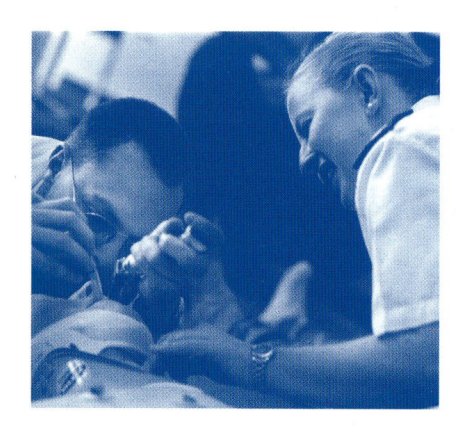

The starting point

9.1 The NHS spends more than £1,000 every second. The Government will introduce new arrangements to ensure that NHS cash is spent wisely and effectively. NHS money will flow around the system in a way that supports quality and efficiency. Such a change will be welcomed by both managers and clinicians. They have struggled with a financial system under the internal market that proved chaotic and costly to run.

9.2 In the internal market, NHS Trusts received their funding under annually negotiated contracts with 100 Health Authorities and some 3,500 GP fundholding groups. Many treatments were individually funded on a 'cost-per-case' or 'extra-contractual-referral' basis. The arrangements were built around adversarial negotiations on the cost and volume of services, with little room left to address quality and outcomes.

'NHS money will flow around the system to support quality and efficiency'

9.3 The financial regime for NHS Trusts, constructed on a quasi-commercial model, encouraged them to compete for marginal extra income. Health Authorities and GPs, for their part, were expected to attempt to shop around for the 'best buy'. Some family doctors had control over some parts of their budgets but some did not. The result was short-termism that prevented the NHS from planning sensibly for change. Nor did the internal market system prove to be financially disciplined or efficient as record financial deficits and administrative costs both demonstrated.

How the money will flow

9.4 The NHS needs funding arrangements which reflect the long-term interdependence of local communities and their local health service, which bring clinicians together to plan improvements over sensible timescales, and which encourage real efficiency as a means to a fair and high quality service.

> *'encourage real efficiency as a means to a fair and high quality service'*

Funding quality and efficiency

The new financial arrangements will promote access to high **quality care** right across the country by:

- fairly distributing resources through Health Authorities to inclusive Primary Care Groups

- establishing new unified budgets for Primary Care Groups covering hospital and community services, GP prescribing and the general practice infrastructure

- allowing clinicians to influence the use of resources by aligning clinical and financial responsibilities

Promote **efficiency** in all areas of NHS activity by:

- offering greater stability and incentives through long-term agreements between Health Authorities, Primary Care Groups and NHS Trusts

- bearing down on costs through benchmarking and a new schedule of national 'reference costs'

- removing the perverse incentives of the market

- reducing bureaucracy by abolishing the internal market.

Fairness

9.5 The Government will raise spending on the NHS in real terms every year and a greater proportion of every pound spent will go on patient care not bureaucracy. In England, the Government has already delivered on this commitment by making available an extra £1 billion for the NHS in 1998-99, and an extra £269 million in 1997-98 to tackle immediate winter pressures and begin the task of modernising

> *'raising spending on the NHS in real terms every year, with more of every pound going on patient care'*

the NHS for the long term. Meantime the stream of action to abolish the internal market, culminating in this White Paper, is already redeploying resources to patient services.

'new mechanisms to distribute NHS cash more fairly'

9.6 The Government will put in place new mechanisms to distribute NHS cash more fairly. A new Advisory Committee on Resource Allocation will further improve the arrangements for distributing resources for both primary and secondary care. The healthcare needs of populations, including the impact of deprivation, will be the driving force in determining where cash goes. There will be a national formula to set fair shares for the new Primary Care Groups, as there is now for Health Authorities. It will be for Health Authorities to determine the pace of change at which individual Primary Care Groups within their area should move towards their fair share. Regional Offices will monitor progress.

'the biggest new hospital building programme in the history of the NHS'

9.7 The Government is putting in place new arrangements to ensure that health service need is the key determinant of funding major capital development in the NHS. This process began with the prioritisation of major acute sector Private Finance Initiative (PFI) schemes. The inherited logjam in PFI has now been broken. The result - the biggest new hospital building programme in the history of the NHS. The Government is establishing a Capital Prioritisation Advisory Group to assess which major capital development projects should proceed. We are also exploring the potential of extending public - private partnerships into non-acute areas, such as information technology and community health services.

Flexibility

'freed from the constraints imposed by artificially distinct budget headings'

9.8 The Government will give clinicians greater control and flexibility over the resources they receive. That means unifying into a single stream of funds three currently separate budgets - for hospital and community health services; family health services prescribing; and cash limited funding for GP practice staff, premises and computers. In the future there will be one stream of cash-limited funds flowing through Health Authorities to Primary Care Groups. That will give GPs the maximum choice about the treatment option that best suits individual patients, free from the constraints imposed by artificially distinct budget headings. It will align clinical and financial responsibility so that those who prescribe, treat and refer have control over the financial decisions they make.

9.9 Within the new framework, the NHS will ensure that all patients have proper access to the medicines they need. The large number of GPs who already have local prescribing budgets have demonstrated the patient care advantages of giving family doctors financial responsibility for their prescribing decisions. The NHS Executive will put in hand work with all the interested players to prepare for a smooth transition to these new arrangements.

'the NHS will ensure that all patients have proper access to the medicines they need'

9.10 It is equally important to integrate health and social care resources so that patients genuinely get access to seamless services. There are already initiatives in place that channel both health and social care funding to provide a single service for patients. The Government will build on these developments. In 1998, we will consult on ways in which still closer relationships at working level, including joint operation and planning of budgets, might help break down traditional barriers and promote a better service for users and carers. We will require joint investment plans from 1999-2000 for continuing care and community care services.

Stability

9.11 In the new NHS, the short-termism of the market will be replaced by a more stable framework based on longer-term relationships. Locally the Health Improvement Programme will set a shared context - within which Health Authorities, Primary Care Groups and NHS Trusts will reach long-term agreements. These agreements will last for at least three years, but could extend in some circumstances for five to ten years, if that was the appropriate time horizon for implementing a programme of development and change.

'a stable framework based on longer term relationships'

9.12 Renewal of agreements will be dependent on satisfactory progress against local objectives, including both cost and quality targets. Primary Care Groups will be able to signal if they wish to make a change either in the nature of the agreement, or in the service provider they use, within the context of the Health Improvement Programme.

9.13 If there are problems with performance, the first step will be for the Primary Care Group and the NHS Trust to explore the difficulty and plan to put it right. The long term agreement could link an element of future payment to satisfactory progress. If there are serious

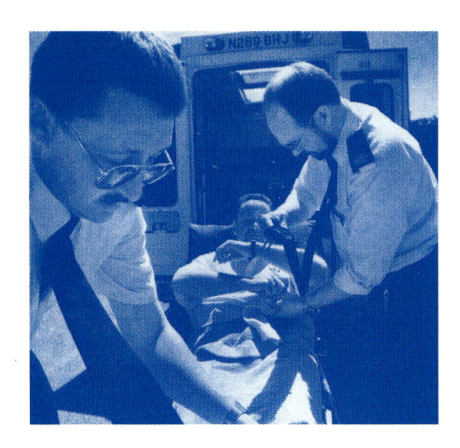

Long-term agreements

- will focus on service delivery objectives, with primary and secondary care clinicians coming together to develop better integrated patterns of care

- address health and quality objectives, as well as cost and volume, reflecting the new rounded approach to performance

- increasingly focus on 'programmes of care' for the population, and pathways for patients that cross traditional organisational boundaries

- recognise that NHS Trusts must share responsibility for ensuring activity does not get out of kilter with funding.

- provide for the benefits of greater efficiency to be shared between the commissioner, on behalf of the community, and the NHS Trust, for investment consistent with the Health Improvement Programme

- contain incentives for improvement, with funding conditional in part on satisfactory progress against key targets

concerns over clinical quality that cannot be resolved locally it will be possible to seek help from the Commission for Health Improvement. If the problem is still not resolved, or there are other reasons to press for change, the Primary Care Group will need to give due notice of the intended change, and to explore its plans with the Health Authority and other users of the service. In this way crucial services for some users will not be destabilised by the actions of others.

9.14 Long-term agreements will replace the annual contracts of the internal market, which wasted so much time, effort and resources throughout the NHS. They will increasingly reflect dialogue between clinicians in primary and secondary care, rather than purely between managers. They will be based around specific services - linked where appropriate to the new National Service Frameworks - rather than whole hospitals. The move away from the annual round to a pattern in which a number of agreements are due for renewal each year will make it possible to look in more depth at service issues and to engage clinicians in planning for improvements over a sensible time horizon.

9.15 To help develop the new approach, the NHS Executive will work with the NHS to assemble a range of default model agreements which local players could use. The aim will be to share good practice as it develops, while minimising unnecessary duplication of local management and clinical effort.

9.16 The combination of new high-level commissioning arrangements for specialist services (as outlined in chapter 7), and long-term agreements which reflect the views of all local GPs, should ensure that all but a small minority of GP referrals to hospitals are covered by these new agreements. On occasion, however, a patient's special clinical needs or personal circumstances will require a GP to make individualised arrangements. It is important that the new system should allow for such cases, but without the bureaucracy associated with the old style 'extra contractual referrals' (ECRs) of the internal market.

9.17 In the ECR system, patients could often find themselves the subject of heated debate between GPs, Trusts and Health Authorities about whether they were covered by a 'contract' and, if not, whether their care would be paid for. These arrangements added substantially to the bureaucracy of the internal market. The ECR system will be abolished and replaced by simplified arrangements that minimise bureaucracy and eliminate incentives to 'play the market'. A new system will be introduced, based on adjustments to Primary Care Group and Health Authority allocations, rather than invoicing. This will align clinical and financial responsibility, coupling the freedom to refer with the ability to fund. The NHS Executive will issue guidance on the details of implementation by summer 1998, to enable new arrangements to be put in place from April 1999.

'ECR system will be abolished'

Efficiency

9.18 Efficient use of resources will be critical to delivering the best for patients. It is important that managers and clinicians alike have a proper understanding of the costs of local services, so that they can make appropriate local decisions on the best use of resources.

9.19 The pricing arrangements of the market have proved complex, time-consuming, and ultimately unsuccessful in driving efficiency. A more transparent approach is needed. Priorities and performance in the NHS have been distorted by an obsession with measuring changes in the 'Purchaser Efficiency Index' without the same regard for improvements in other areas. Quality has suffered and incentives to increase activity have flown in the face of effective financial management. The old style Purchaser Efficiency Index will be replaced by demanding and better measures of efficiency by 1 April 1999. Chapter 8 has set out plans for a new, balanced approach to assessing the NHS's performance against the things that count most for patients, setting new measures of efficiency within a wider context.

'a programme which requires NHS Trusts to publish and benchmark their costs on a consistent basis'

9.20 The new approach will include demanding targets on unit cost and productivity throughout the NHS. The Government will develop a programme which requires NHS Trusts to publish and benchmark their costs on a consistent basis. This will provide a national schedule of 'reference costs' which will itemise the cost of individual treatments across the NHS. Costs for major areas of hospital activity will be available in time to inform long-term agreements for 1999-2000.

> *'bearing down on costs to achieve best value'*

9.21 Where the schedule indicates poor performance, Health Authorities, Primary Care Groups and NHS Trusts will need to investigate why, sort out plans to tackle inefficiencies, and build these into long-term agreements. Primary Care Groups will be expected to bear down on NHS Trusts costs over time so as to achieve best possible value for their local community. Where NHS Trusts prove unable to make satisfactory progress over a period of time, the Regional Office will investigate and, if necessary, intervene.

9.22 This new approach replaces the internal market mechanisms with a stronger national drive, consistent with other action to promote comparative information. The new cost data will be made available to the public alongside other data on NHS Trust performance. Over time, this approach will be developed to support the formation of long-term agreements built around programmes of care for patients with different needs, rather than individual treatments.

Cutting bureaucracy

> *'this White Paper, by completing the abolition of the internal market, will release further resources from bureaucracy'*

9.23 When it came into office, the Government began the process of dismantling the internal market. In the process it has cut unnecessary red tape and shifted resources into patient care. This White Paper, by completing the abolition of the internal market, will release further resources from bureaucracy.

9.24 NHS Trust management costs will be cut, as a result of reduced transactions, the abolition of ECRs, and progressive improvements in efficiency as part of the drive to improved and more consistent performance. Health Authority costs will be cut, through measures to improve efficiency, to share and streamline core functions, and to reduce administration and transaction costs. Removing the bureaucracy of GP fundholding (which covered only a minority of hospital and community services for half the population) will make it possible to support Primary Care Groups covering all services across the whole of the population while containing expenditure to a level below that planned by the previous Government for fundholding administration in 1997-98.

9.25 In total, £1 billion will be freed up from bureaucracy for patient care over the lifetime of the Parliament. Activities that served the bureaucracy of the market will be stripped away. Future arrangements for measuring and monitoring management costs will reflect the new approach. A modern NHS will need strong leadership, committed to ensuring that all management activity supports the core purpose of improving health and health care.

> *'£1 billion will be freed up from bureaucracy for patient care'*

Cutting bureaucracy

The Government's action to end the internal market will cut bureaucracy by:

- replacing the annual contract round with long-term agreements

- abolishing ECRs and cost-per-case contracts

- moving from GP fundholding to inclusive Primary Care Groups

- reshaping Health Authorities with savings in core administrative functions to allow reinvestment in their new role

- ending competition and bearing down on NHS Trust management and administrative costs generated by the internal market

- integrating primary care and community trusts, and sharing support functions between NHS organisations.

Milestones

1998

- consultation on steps to improve joint working between health and social care
- first tranche of long-term agreements
- publication of NHS Trusts costs and the schedule of 'reference costs'

1999

- introduction of new combined HCHS, GP prescribing and cash-limited GMS budgets from April 1999

10

Key themes

- *building on what works*
- *Health Action Zones to blaze the trail*
- *a rolling programme of development*

Making it happen
rolling out change

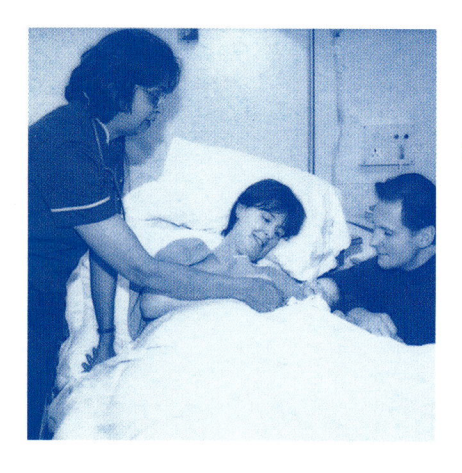

Modernising the NHS

10.1 This White Paper marks a watershed for the NHS. It sets a clear direction for the NHS as a modern and dependable service. But it will not mean a wholesale structural upheaval, generating costs and disruption that get in the way of patient care. The NHS has had all too much of that. There is no appetite amongst patients or staff for such an upheaval. But there is an appetite for change that goes with the grain of the NHS and its traditional values.

'a clear direction for the NHS as a modern and dependable service'

10.2 Indeed the NHS has to change. It has to modernise to meet the demands of a new century. The modernisation programme outlined in this White Paper provides the means to deliver easier, faster access to more consistent and higher quality care for patients. Although it cannot all be achieved at once, some improvement will begin immediately. The Government wants to see the NHS getting better every year.

10.3 We have already made a start with early action on each of the themes in this White Paper:

- action to raise standards across the country in breast cancer services and paediatric care, in a **single national** health service

'the NHS getting better every year'

- announcement of new Health Action Zones to explore **new, flexible, local** ways of delivering health and healthcare

- a new approach to **partnership** in the NHS for the 1998-99 commissioning round

- action to improve **efficiency** by reducing management costs

- action teams to tackle inherited rising waiting lists and times, improving **performance** across the country

- rebuilding **public confidence** by opening NHS Trust Board meetings to the public and launching consultation on a new NHS Charter.

10.4 The Government will work closely with those in the NHS, users and carers, and partner organisations on implementation. There will be early consultation papers on some issues. Others will be taken forward locally, but with arrangements to identify and share good practice as it develops. In parallel, the NHS Executive will work with the health service locally to promote the organisational and personal development that must support clinicians and managers as they put these new arrangements in place and respond to the new challenges.

'a rolling programme of modernisation'

10.5 Early steps will be taken to clear out of the way the obstacles created by the internal market and put in place some building blocks - for example the new Primary Care Groups, and new Institute and Commission to drive the new focus on quality. The chart at the end of the chapter sets out the early milestones. The main new components of the systems set out in this White Paper will, subject to the availability of Parliamentary time for the necessary legislation, be in place and operational by 1999.

10.6 New Health Action Zones will blaze the trail. Starting in up to ten areas from April 1998, they will bring together all those in a Health Authority area or wider, to improve the health of local people. The accent will be on partnership and innovation, finding new ways to tackle health problems and reshape local services. Health Action Zones will be concentrated in areas of pronounced deprivation and poor health, reflecting the Government's commitment to tackle entrenched inequalities. An early task for each Health Action Zone will be to develop clear targets, agreed with the NHS Executive, for measurable improvements every year.

'Health Action Zones will blaze the trail'

10.7 The same process of planning and delivering measurable improvements year by year must apply throughout the NHS, nationally and locally. Our programme will develop a new 24 hour nurse-led advice line, reduced waiting times for patients with suspected cancer, and better services in the community through the NHS's own information superhighway. They will all provide faster, modern, reliable services for patients. The forthcoming Green Paper *Our Healthier Nation* will consult on new national targets for promoting better health. We are already consulting on a new NHS Charter to be published in 1998. The new NHS performance framework will help target further areas for improvement, both nationally and locally.

> *'an NHS that responds to a changed and changing world'*

10.8 This is a tough and challenging programme. On some fronts there will be early progress. Others may be for the long haul. Some may take time to show visible improvement. But the end result will be an NHS that responds to a changed and changing world. Where patients can expect services to be quickly available of consistently high quality. Where medical advance can be harnessed and made more locally available. Where care is there for people when they need it, where they need it. An NHS that is accessible and responsive. An NHS which gets better every year. A modern and dependable NHS.

Making it happen

Early Milestones

1998

- three telephone advice helplines set up

- projects established to demonstrate benefits of NHS' own information superhighway

- new Information Management and Technology Strategy for the NHS published

- consultation documents on quality and performance issued

- Public Health Green Paper *Our Healthier Nation* issued

- Health Action Zones begin

- new NHS Charter

- first survey of users and carers

- Health Authorities begin work with partner organisations on prototype Health Improvement Programmes for the period beginning 1999-2000

- GP Commissioning Pilots begin

- development work on Primary Care Groups, on new financial arrangements, and on new performance indicators

1999

(Precise timing subject to legislation)

- two week waiting time for urgent suspected breast cancer cases

- new Primary Care Groups begin, subsuming GP fundholding

- new statutory duties on partnership, health and quality

- development of local clinical governance, the new National Institute for Clinical Excellence and Commission for Health Improvement

- new unified local health budgets for hospital and community services, GP prescribing and the general practice infrastructure

- new funding arrangements for NHS Trusts in place

Annex
Primary Care Trusts

1. The Government will establish a new form of Trust - the Primary Care Trust - for Primary Care Groups which wish to be independent and are capable of being so. The Government will issue detailed proposals for discussion in due course, but such Trusts could be managed by a board of GPs (drawn from the practices involved), community nurses and managers, and include social services and lay members. The Trust would hold the resources for General Medical Services cash-limited allocations, hospital and community health services and prescribing. One option would be for the Trust to hold a wider range of resources under the so-called 'unified budget' option under the Primary Care Act. GPs who wished to retain their existing independent contractor status under Part II of the (1977) NHS Act would do so.

2. Community health services, and in many cases the NHS Trusts which provide them, will have an important part to play in contributing to the work of Primary Care Groups in commissioning services and in integrating their provision with that of primary care. There will be scope, where a Primary Care Trust is established, for appropriate community health services and their management to become an integral part of the Trust.

3. In such cases it is envisaged that the Primary Care Trust will employ all relevant community health staff and run community hospitals and other community facilities, ensuring these work effectively as part of an integrated system. The precise arrangements will, however, depend on local circumstances.

4. The new Trusts will not be expected to take responsibility for specialised mental health or learning disability services.

5. The Government envisages that the criteria for a Primary Care Group to become independent would include:

    - proper arrangements for financial accountability, including the appointment of the Chair or Chief Executive as the Accountable Officer, and arrangements to ensure the Trust balances its budget and meets its cash limit

- well developed arrangements for monitoring activity and developing practice-level clinical standards

- making an effective contribution and working within the Health Improvement Programme set by the Health Authority and partner organisations

- agreed standards and targets set with the Health Authority

- broad support locally for the establishment of such a Trust, including amongst those GPs affected.

Primary Care Trusts will be accountable to the local Health Authority.

The Government will evaluate early progress with these arrangements before enabling them to evolve generally.

Glossary

Acute Services
Medical and surgical treatment and care mainly provided in hospitals.

Calman-Hine Cancer Report
The report *A Policy Framework for Commissioning Cancer Services* which was commissioned in response to concerns about variations in treatment across the country. It recommended that cancer services should be organised at three levels: primary care; cancer units in local hospitals with multi-disciplinary teams able to treat the commoner cancers; and cancer centres situated in larger hospitals to treat the less common cancers and support cancer units with services such as radiotherapy, not available in smaller hospitals.

Capital
Capital expenditure is spending on the acquisition of land and premises, and on the provision, adaption, renewal, replacement or demolition of buildings, items or groups of equipment and vehicles etc where the expenditure exceeds £5,000.

Cash Limit
The amount of money the Government proposes to spend or authorise on certain services or blocks of services during one financial year.

Clinical Governance
A new initiative in this White Paper (chapter 6) to assure and improve clinical standards at local level throughout the NHS. This includes action to ensure that risks are avoided, adverse events are rapidly detected, openly investigated and lessons learned, good practice is rapidly disseminated and systems are in place to ensure continuous improvements in clinical care.

Clinician
A health professional who is directly involved in the care and treatment of patients, for example nurses, doctors, therapists, midwives.

Commission for Health Improvement

A new national body proposed in this White Paper to support and oversee the quality of clinical governance and of clinical services.

Community Health Councils

Independent statutory bodies which were established in 1974 and represent the interests of the public in the health service in their area.

Community Nurses

Includes practice nurses, district nurses, health visitors, school nurses.

Extra Contractual Referrals (ECRs)

An arrangement under the NHS internal market to cover a referral to an NHS Trust for which there was no existing contract with the patient's Health Authority of residence or GP fundholder.

General Medical Services

General medical services are services provided by family doctors (GPs) and their staff, as provided for in Section 29 of the 1997 Act, and framed in the General Medical Services Regulations 1992.

GP Commissioning Groups

Pilot projects preparing to go live from April 1998. Based around groups of fundholding and non-fundholding GPs. Will manage a prescribing budget. Will work closely with their local Health Authority to develop health strategies and advise on service developments for local populations.

GP Fundholding

A GP whose practice manages a budget for its practice staff, certain hospital referrals, drug costs, community nursing services and management costs.

Health Action Zones

A new initiative to bring together organisations within and beyond the NHS to develop and implement a locally agreed strategy for improving the health of local people. Up to 10 Zones, generally covering an area of at least Health Authority size, will be selected to go live from April 1998.

Health Authority

Chapter 4 sets out the role and responsibilities of Health Authorities within the new NHS.

Health Improvement Programmes

An action programme to improve health and healthcare locally and led by the Health Authority. Will involve NHS Trusts, Primary Care Groups, other primary care professionals, working in partnership with the local authority and engaging other local interests. See chapter 4.

Hospital and Community Health Services (HCHS)

The main elements of these are the provision of hospital services, and certain community health services, such as district nursing. These services are provided in the main by NHS Trusts.

Local Medical Committee

The statutory Local Representative Committee for all GPs in the area covered by a Health Authority. The Health Authority has a statutory duty to consult it on issues including GPs' terms of service, complaints and the investigation of certain matters of professional conduct.

Long-Term Service Agreements

Agreements between Health Authorities or Primary Care Groups and NHS Trusts on the service to be provided for a local population. These replace the annual contracts of the internal market and cover a minimum of three years to offer greater stability. See chapter 9.

Multifunds

Groups of GP fundholders who agree to pool their budgets and work together.

National Institute of Clinical Excellence

A new Institute which will be set up to promote clinical and cost-effectiveness and the production and dissemination of clinical guidelines. See chapter 7.

National Schedule of Reference Costs

NHS Trusts will be required to publish their costs on a consistent basis, and the data published in a national schedule of 'reference costs' so that performance on efficiency can be benchmarked. See chapter 9.

National Service Frameworks

National Service Frameworks will bring together the best evidence of clinical and cost-effectiveness with the views of service users to determine the best ways of providing particular services. See chapter 7.

NHS Executive
The NHS Executive is part of the Department of Health, with offices in London and Leeds and eight Regional Offices across the country (see below). It supports Ministers and provides leadership and a range of central management functions to the NHS.

NHS Trusts
NHS Trusts are public bodies providing NHS hospital and community healthcare.

Performance Framework
The Government will shortly be publishing a consultation document on the new national performance framework set out in this new White Paper. The framework is designed to give a rounded picture of NHS performance and will cover six areas: health improvement; fair access to services; effective delivery of appropriate healthcare; efficiency; patient/carer experience; and the health outcomes of NHS care. See chapter 8.

Personal Medical Services Primary Care Act Pilots
The NHS (Primary Care) Act 1997 allows members of the NHS 'family', ie: an NHS Trust, an NHS employee, a qualifying body and suitably experienced medical practitioners capable of providing general medical services to submit proposals to provide services under a pilot scheme and contract with the Health Authority to do so.
Note: Personal Medical Services are the same types of services that are currently known as General Medical Services.

Personal Social Services
Personal care services for vulnerable people, including those with special needs because of old age or physical or mental disability, and children in need of care and protection. Examples are residential care homes for the elderly, home help and home care services, and social workers who provide help and support for a wide range of people. Local authorities have the statutory responsibilities for them.

Practice Fund Management Allowance
The public money paid to GPs to meet the extra administrative costs of running a fundholding scheme.

Primary Care
Family health services provided by family doctors, dentists, pharmacists, optometrists and ophthalmic medical practitioners.

Glossary

Primary Care Groups

These new Groups, announced in this White Paper, will bring together family doctors and community nurses. They will contribute to the local Health Improvement Programme and have a budget reflecting their population's share of the available resources for hospital and community health services, the general medical services cash limited budget, and prescribing. These Groups will have the opportunity to become freestanding Primary Care Trusts.
See chapter 5.

Regional Offices

See NHS Executive.

Revenue

Expenditure other than capital. For example, staff salaries, drug budgets, etc.

Secondary Care

Specialist care, typically provided in a hospital setting or following referral from a primary or community health professional.

Total Purchasing Projects

Total purchasers comprise groups of GPs who together purchase hospital and community care services not covered by the fundholding scheme on behalf of their patients, working closely with the Health Authority. Legal responsibility for these services remains with the relevant Health Authority.

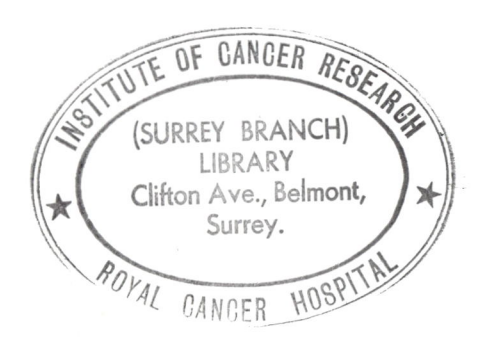